A Woman's Guide to Living with Heart Disease

A Woman's Guide to Living with Heart Disease

Carolyn Thomas

Foreword by Martha Gulati, MD, FACC

WITHDRAWN

Johns Hopkins University Press

Baltimore

Note to the Reader: This book is not meant to substitute for medical care and treatment should not be based solely on its contents. Instead, treatment must be developed in a dialogue between the individual and her or his physician. This book has been written to help with that dialogue.

© 2017 Johns Hopkins University Press
All rights reserved. Published 2017
Printed in the United States of America on acid-free paper
2 4 6 8 9 7 5 3 1

Johns Hopkins University Press
2715 North Charles Street
Baltimore, Maryland 21218-4363
www.press.jhu.edu

Library of Congress Cataloging-in-Publication Data

Names: Thomas, Carolyn, 1950–, author.
Title: A woman's guide to living with heart disease / Carolyn Thomas.
Description: Baltimore : Johns Hopkins University Press, 2017. |
Includes bibliographical references and index.
Identifiers: LCCN 2017009948 | ISBN 9781421424194 (hardcover) |
ISBN 1421424193 (hardcover) | ISBN 9781421424200 (paperback) |
ISBN 1421424207 (paperback) | ISBN 9781421424217 (electronic) |
ISBN 1421424215 (electronic)
Subjects: LCSH: Heart diseases in women. | BISAC: HEALTH & FITNESS /
Diseases / Heart. | MEDICAL / Public Health. | HEALTH & FITNESS /
Women's Health.
Classification: LCC RC682 .T53 2017 | DDC 616.1/20082—dc23
LC record available at https://lccn.loc.gov/2017009948

A catalog record for this book is available from the British Library.

*Special discounts are available for bulk purchases of this book. For more information,
please contact Special Sales at 410-516-6936 or specialsales@press.jhu.edu.*

Johns Hopkins University Press uses environmentally friendly book materials, including
recycled text paper that is composed of at least 30 percent post-consumer waste,
whenever possible.

To my darling grandbaby, Everly Rose.

On the day you were born,
one of my *Heart Sisters* blog readers predicted,
"This precious little child will do more good
for your heart than anything your cardiologist
could ever prescribe for you."

She was right.

Contents

Foreword

We cannot change what we are not aware of, and once we are aware, we cannot help but change.

Sheryl Sandberg, *Lean In: Women, Work, and the Will to Lead*

The good physician treats the disease; the great physician treats the patient who has the disease.

Sir William Osler, 1st Baronet, MDCM, FRS, FRCP

As a young medical student at the University of Toronto in Canada, I became acutely aware of the differences in how we treated men and women who presented with a heart attack. The symptoms of men were never doubted. If a man mentioned chest pain or chest pressure, a heart attack was always the first on the list of potential causes of what was going on, and the hospital team rushed to determine if the man was having a heart attack and take the next steps. Time was heart muscle! It was understood that this was the number-one killer of men. With women, I watched doctors ask more questions about the chest pain: "What is going on at home, Mrs. Jones?"; "Are you under some stress, Ms. Smith?"; "What did you eat today, Ms. Black?" The sense of urgency was rarely seen. Even when a woman had classic symptoms of a heart attack, rather than rushing to get an ECG or taking her straight to the cardiac cath lab, I saw doctors delay the treatment to make sure stress, anxiety, or reflux was not the cause of her symptoms. This delay, despite the fact that heart disease was also the number-one killer of women.

This behavior shocked me, because I was very aware that heart disease and strokes had taken the lives of women in my family. I became convinced that women's symptoms were taken less seriously by doctors, and the emerging evidence at the time supported that conclusion.

Women who had heart attacks were less likely to get guideline-recommended therapies, less likely to receive timely care, less likely to undergo any revascularization, and more likely to die than men. I began to think about what would happen to me, my sister, my cousins, and my girlfriends. What would happen to us if we ultimately had a heart attack? Why would we, just because we are women, be treated so differently? Suddenly I knew what my mission had to be: I was going to have to be a cardiologist who cared exclusively for women and who studied heart disease in women, if I was to be part of the change.

I have now had the honor and privilege to care for women and their hearts for many years. And I hope I have been part of the change in caring for women. Nonetheless, we are still at the infancy of understanding women's hearts and the impact of heart disease on the lives of women affected by this disease. It remains both of interest and of concern to me that heart disease is still underappreciated both by women and by physicians.

Additionally, it remains a "secret disease" for many women; unlike breast cancer, heart disease is rarely discussed, despite the enormity of the disease and its impact on women. The perception that a woman is to be blamed for a heart attack is one of many reasons women are often silent after a heart attack, despite the fact that many risk factors for heart disease overlap with risk factors for breast cancer. It still is often thought of as a man's disease despite all the marketing, education, and public awareness campaigns driven toward educating women about their risk of the greatest killer.

We continue to see gender gaps in the treatment and management of heart disease and stroke, with persistently worse outcomes and higher mortality in women, particularly younger women, compared to men. We continue to have gender gaps in the enrollment of women in cardiovascular trials. Only recently was it mandated that cellular research and animal studies include both sexes, where again, the female sex has often been excluded. So there is much more work to do in both helping women understand that they are at risk for heart disease, as well as improving the education of physicians in order to close this gender gap in heart disease outcomes. And further, we need to continue to advocate for more research to be done on women and their hearts so we can become better at preventing and treating heart disease in women.

A Woman's Guide to Living with Heart Disease is an excellent book that will not only benefit any woman living with heart disease, but also physicians and other health professionals caring for women. It gives a unique perspective on heart disease that has really not been heard until now—the patient's perspective. Carolyn Thomas is a woman who lives with heart disease. As a result of her personal experience, she has become the voice of many patients in the world through her blog, her writings, her public speaking, and now through this book. As a woman who experienced a heart attack, was misdiagnosed, and deals with everything that living with heart disease entails, Carolyn uses humor wrapped in practicality and common sense to help women navigate their disease and all the overwhelming emotions that come with this diagnosis. Additionally, she has provided useful information for health care teams to appreciate what patients need and expect from their practitioners. To paraphrase the above quote from Osler, the great physician will treat not just the disease but the patient. As a physician, I feel that that is also the message Carolyn sends to us. And it is an important one for the health care team to remember.

I have had the pleasure of knowing Carolyn, first through her writings and then eventually in person. Our bond was threefold: our mutual love of the heart, our desire to make sure (she as a laywoman, I as a doctor) that medical information was fully and accurately translated to patients living with heart disease and—last but not least—our love for our homeland, Canada. I am so grateful to have her as someone I send my patients to connect with on the Internet. Her thoughtful comments on her experiences, combined with her interviews of others and her reflections on research, have made her the voice of the heart patient. Hers is the voice I hear when I look at my patient and realize that everything I said was not absorbed because my patient is still recoiling from the diagnosis I handed her. She is the person whispering in my ear, asking me to remember to introduce everyone in the room. She (and her blog) is the reason I insisted that the gowns in my women's heart center open in the front and are warm and cozy.

Carolyn has given a voice to the female heart patient in a way that few others have been able to. I am grateful that she decided to write this book, because I believe it will improve the dialogue between heart patients and their physicians. She empowers women to improve their health, their life, and their ability to communicate with their doctors effectively. She also validates what many patients feel but have not been able to express. This book will allow women living with heart disease to know they are not alone and, I hope, will help them find their own voices.

Martha Gulati, MD, FACC
Editor-in-Chief, CardioSmart, American College of Cardiology
Chief of Cardiology, University of Arizona
Author of *Saving Women's Hearts: How You Can Prevent and Reverse Heart Disease with Natural and Conventional Strategies*

Preface

The ink was barely dry on the book contract I'd signed with Johns Hopkins University Press on the morning I tuned in, as I like to do every weekend, to Michael Enright's *Sunday Edition* show on CBC Radio. Michael's guest that morning couldn't have been more appropriate, given the project I was just beginning. A physician-turned-author named Dr. Suzanne Koven was talking about people who write first-person accounts of their health crises, books that Michael indelicately referred to as "sick lit."[1]

Illness, he began, is always more interesting to the ill person than to the reader. But Dr. Koven quickly interjected. It's possible, she insisted, to "write about your own experience of illness in a way that's not only informative about the illness for a general audience, but in a way that speaks to broader human questions." The illness narrative, she added, isn't just about illness, "but can also be about big themes like identity and life and death and love and resilience."

Then Michael suggested that the most popular illness narratives surely must come from those living with cancer or with an addiction to drugs or alcohol. "You need high stakes to make a good story, don't you?" Cancer and addiction certainly provide those stakes, he added, because we associate both with the ultimate threat to life.

Dr. Koven interjected again, this time wondering aloud why heart disease has not been a more prominent book theme for survivors to address, especially when you consider what she called "the metaphorical resonance of the heart" and the fact that heart disease is one of our most deadly health threats, killing more women every year than all forms of cancer combined.

Why, she asked, aren't we seeing a lot of books written by heart patients?

I asked that same question myself eight years earlier as a freshly diagnosed heart attack survivor. I wasn't looking for books about cardiac risk factors or heart-healthy recipes or bad cholesterol. What I desperately wanted to find were books written for and by women like me.

The book you're holding now is the one I couldn't find back then when I really needed it.

I'm not a physician. I'm not a scientist (although I spent two decades living with one—does that count at all?). As I often describe myself, I'm just a dull-witted heart attack survivor. But I'm also a woman who, like far too many others, had her heart disease misdiagnosed. There's nothing quite like a misdiagnosis to heighten the high stakes required to make a good story.

After graduating from the Mayo Clinic training program called the WomenHeart Science and Leadership Symposium in 2008, I taught myself how to figure out cardiac research papers published in medical journals. And then I translated those studies into plain English for my *Heart Sisters* blog readers.[2] In 2014, the *British Medical Journal (BMJ)* invited me to join their team of patient reviewers for cardiology papers submitted to the journal for publication. And when the Vancouver Coastal Health Research Foundation invited me to speak at a public forum on women's heart disease, they later described me as a "knowledge translator."[3] I love that job description!

I have learned that, as Dr. Suzanne Koven assured Michael Enright's radio audience, in my story and in the stories I share about other women (no matter what their diagnoses), readers appear eager to see—and are in fact responding to—what she calls those "big themes." They are indeed as important to us as the diagnosis itself.

None of us can ever truly prepare for how a catastrophic medical crisis can change our lives and those of our loved ones. While navigating our way, we could use an experienced, trustworthy friend alongside who's traveled the same road before us. My hope is that, in reading this book, you will find that companion.

Acknowledgments

Thank you to those who have visited my *Heart Sisters* blog since I launched the site in 2009, to those who have shared your brilliant, funny, heartbreaking, or provocative comments with me, and to those who have trusted me to tell your story, because those stories deserve to be known. You are my tribe, and you remind me every day that I'm not alone.

Thank you to the thousands of women (and a few men!) who continue to surprise me by filling my Heart-Smart Women presentation audiences (or sitting patiently on waiting lists to get in). And special thanks to the visionary physicians who have embraced the Patients Included movement by inviting people like me to share the patient perspective at your medical conferences.

Thank you to Dr. Sharonne Hayes at Mayo Clinic for your pioneering accomplishments in transforming ordinary heart patients into trained activists and educators "gunning for bear" (as you like to say). Your contagious passion, demonstrated while leading the annual WomenHeart Science and Leadership Symposium (Mayo class of 2008), changed my life.

Thank you to my favorite daughter-in-law, Paula Dunn, for your sharp eye and legendary proofreading skills, and for cheerfully devoting countless hours (mostly, it seems, spent proofing hard copies on the treadmill during your lunch breaks, or reviewing online copy at 2:30 a.m. while the rest of us slept) in order to help make this a better book. I owe you brunch at Cora's, and so much more.

Thank you to Jackie Wehmueller, former executive editor at Johns Hopkins University Press, for convincing me that your vision of a blog-turned-book could become my vision, too. And thanks also to JHUP senior production editor Deborah Bors for your copyediting skills and your kindness when I most needed both.

Living with heart disease has been made so much easier for me than I know it is for many others because of the truly remarkable physicians who have cared for and about me, including Dr. Manjeet Mann, Dr. Nelson Svorkdal, Dr. Kate Whittaker, and Dr. Marie Skinnider. I appreciate every one of you.

Thank you so much to my family and friends. Your love and laughter, as always, have made the bad days bearable and the good days delicious.

A Woman's Guide to Living with Heart Disease

1 ♡ The First Signs

"This better not be a heart attack. Because I do not have time for this!"

Those are my first thoughts as I lean heavily against the Garry oak tree, surveying my shocking circumstances. It's early, barely sunrise, even too early on this quiet spring day for dog walkers or Monday morning commuters heading for the bus. So it's just me, alone, on a long leafy block of Belmont Avenue, my right hand clutching that tree trunk.

I'd set out extra early on my walk this morning because I'm delivering a little stack of thank-you notes, popping them quietly into the mailboxes of still-sleeping neighbors and friends who have just helped to celebrate my fifty-eighth birthday the day before.

I try to take stock of what has suddenly stopped my daily walk: central chest pain, a sickening wave of nausea, sweating, and hot prickly pressure radiating down my left arm. I look up and down Belmont to see if I can spot somebody, anybody, who can help me. I'm starting to feel frightened because this chest pain is so intense that I know I can't walk.

Walk? I can hardly breathe.

After what seems like an hour, but is probably closer to just 15 or 20 minutes, I'm relieved to find that my symptoms seem to be easing. After several more minutes, I try taking a few cautious steps away from my Garry oak toward the sidewalk. I walk gingerly, slowly, step by step, heading home just a few blocks away. But as I walk slowly home, it's the trace of that weirdly painful prickle down my arm that still niggles me, because I recall reading or hearing something about left arm pain being a possible sign of a heart attack.

Heart attack!

Heart attack?

It turns out that I'll be walking right past my local hospital on my way home. Maybe I should pop into the Emergency Department while I'm so close by.

"I think I may be having a heart attack." My voice is a barely audible whisper to the ER nurse sitting at the admitting desk. I don't really want to cause a commotion, because right now, those scary symptoms have almost disappeared and I'm already convincing myself that I'm likely just wasting their time. But within seconds, I'm ushered in, lying on a gurney, hooked up to a 12-lead electrocardiogram (EKG), with an IV started in my right hand. Everything is happening so fast. I'm given all the standard cardiac diagnostic tests that current treatment guidelines recommend for any person who presents to the ER with those same textbook heart attack symptoms.

An ER physician approaches my bedside with the first cardiac enzyme blood test results. He's an older doctor (translation: about my age), with clean-cut graying hair, a white coat, and a quick officious manner. He begins asking me questions, but he's looking down at his clipboard taking notes the whole time, and he has not yet introduced himself to me.

"Are you the doctor?" I interrupt him to ask.

Yes, he nods with a pinched frown, but he neither makes eye contact nor volunteers his name. Instead, he tells me that the results of my EKG and the first of two cardiac enzyme blood tests look normal. They'll do a second blood test soon, as the guidelines dictate, but "that one will be normal, too," he predicts confidently.

Before he leaves my bedside, the doctor asks, while scribbling more notes, if I've ever been diagnosed with heartburn or GERD (gastroesophageal reflux disease), because, as he observes, "You are in the right demographic for acid reflux."

No, not even mild indigestion. Ever. I'm the picture of health. Until recent heel injuries, I'd been a distance runner for decades, and I'm practically a vegetarian (except for bacon, of course). I have a busy social life and a public relations job I love at this very hospital's hospice and palliative care unit.

But now I recall that I did have an extra glass or two of wine at my party, plus the over-the-top birthday dinner, and, yes, there was that large piece of delicious homemade cake. Maybe this is just what heartburn or acid reflux feels like after a big birthday party splurge.

When my second normal blood test results are confirmed, the doctor returns and tells me to go home and make an appointment with my family physician, who will prescribe antacid drugs for my stomach problems.

By now, I'm feeling exquisitely embarrassed. I cannot wait to get out of there. I've just made a big fuss over nothing but a simple case of heartburn. I apologize to the staff for wasting their valuable time while all those truly sick people in the ER waiting room have been lined up behind me. "Not a problem," one of the nurses reassures me. "But come back to see us if you get worse."

Before I can leave the hospital, another nurse returns to my bedside to remove assorted lines still attached. She looks down at me on the gurney and issues this stern scolding: "You'll have to stop asking questions of the doctor. He is a very good doctor, and he does not like to be questioned."

Now I'm not only feeling embarrassed, but I'm also humiliated at being spoken to like this. I can feel my cheeks burning hot, as if I were an unruly child threatened with a spanking for being naughty.

And the question I'd had the temerity to ask the doctor?

"But Doc, what about this pain down my left arm?"

The Slow-Onset Heart Attack

There were a number of good reasons I had no trouble believing the ER physician who sent me home with that acid reflux misdiagnosis. These reasons were:

- ♥ He had the letters MD after his name.
- ♥ He diagnosed me in a decisively authoritative manner.
- ♥ I wanted to believe him because I'd much rather have indigestion than heart disease, thank you very much.
- ♥ The ER nurse scolded me about daring to ask a question of this doctor.
- ♥ Most of all, what I had wrongly imagined a heart attack looking like (clutching one's chest in agony, falling down unconscious) was not at all what I was experiencing.

Despite my own alarming symptoms, I was still able to generally behave exactly like I pictured somebody who was not having a heart attack would behave. So it somehow all made sense to me as I was being sent home from the ER that day.

For many patients, however, a heart attack might present as something that researchers in Ireland refer to as *slow-onset MI* (myocardial infarction, or heart attack). Dr. Sharon O'Donnell, lead author of a study published in the *Journal of Cardiovascular Nursing*, explained that slow-onset MI is the gradual onset of symptoms, coming and going over a long period of time,[1] while *fast-onset MI* describes sudden, continuous, and severe heart attack symptoms, particularly chest pain.

More than 60 percent of the study's participants had experienced this slow-onset MI. What all of them had expected, however, were the severe symptoms associated with fast-onset MI, that classic Hollywood heart attack we see portrayed in the media. This mismatch of expected and actual symptoms for participants with slow-onset MI led them to blame their symptoms on a non-cardiac cause as well as to a dangerous treatment-seeking delay.

Study participants who had experienced the more sudden symptoms of a fast-onset MI quickly chalked them up as heart related, which meant making significantly faster decisions to seek immediate medical help.

Typical and Atypical Heart Attack Signs

The frightening symptoms I was experiencing during that eventful early morning walk in May 2008 were what physicians (and Dr. Google) would consider to be classic heart attack signs. My most debilitating symptom at the time was chest pain that doctors know as *angina pectoris* (a Latin name that translates gruesomely as "strangulation of the chest").

Typical heart attack symptoms in both men and women can include:

♥ chest pain or discomfort
♥ nausea
♥ fatigue
♥ shortness of breath

♥ sweating

♥ dizziness

But, particularly in women, *atypical cardiac symptoms* may also be reported. For example:

♥ chest pain, which may be central or be felt armpit to armpit, but *in at least 10 percent of women, no chest symptoms at all are present during a heart attack*[2]

♥ an abrupt change in how your body feels

♥ unusual pain, discomfort, pressure, heaviness, burning, tightness, or fullness in the left or right arm, upper back, shoulder, neck, throat, jaw, or abdomen

♥ weakness, fainting, light-headedness, or extreme/unusual fatigue

♥ shortness of breath and/or difficulty breathing

♥ restlessness, insomnia, or anxiety

♥ a bluish color or numbness in lips, hands, or feet

♥ nausea or vomiting

♥ clammy sweats (or sweating that's out of proportion to your level of exertion or environment)

♥ persistent dry, barking cough

♥ a sense of impending doom

During a heart attack, our heart muscle cells begin to run out of oxygen because something is preventing the oxygenated blood flowing through our coronary arteries from feeding that muscle. A heart attack may also cause a sensation of pain to travel from the heart to the spinal cord, where many nerves merge onto the same nerve pathway. Your arm may be perfectly fine, for example, but your brain thinks that part of your pain is in the arm (or in the jaw, shoulder, elbow, neck, or upper back) screaming out for help. That's what *referred pain* is. It happens when pain is located away from or adjacent to the specific organ involved—such as in a person's jaw or shoulder, but not necessarily anywhere near the chest.

Not all of these signs occur during every cardiac event. Some female survivors report that their symptoms came on suddenly and simply felt unusual rather than alarming. Sometimes the most extreme symptoms don't necessarily imply the worst heart muscle damage. Symptoms can often go away and then return over time. *Stable* symptoms typically become worse with exertion but go away with rest. If symptoms come on when you're at rest, they're considered to be *unstable*—and that could mean a serious emergency for which you need immediate medical care.

There's Pain, and Then There's Pain

I was thinking about the freakish nature of pain recently. When those first alarming warning signs of a heart attack struck me out of the blue, the reality was not what I would have ever imagined a heart attack to feel like. I'd always figured that anybody having a heart attack would clutch dramatically at his chest (in my stereotype, this person was always a man) before crashing down onto the floor, unconscious.

But on that morning, I was fully conscious throughout, and able to walk and talk and think throughout my entire visit to the ER. So really, how could this be a heart attack?

I did not know then, by the way, that my stereotype is not a heart attack at all. Instead, that's called *sudden cardiac arrest* (which is actually a type of electrical problem with the heart, whereas a heart attack is more of a plumbing problem). And yes, men are two to three times more likely to experience sudden cardiac arrest than women are.[3]

Because I was clueless about heart attacks, it was easier for me to believe the ER physician who had sent me home that same morning with an acid reflux misdiagnosis.

At our regional pain clinic, where I've been a regular visitor ever since my heart attack because of what doctors call refractory angina (that's chest pain that's not relieved by usual cardiac treatments), we learn a lot about pain self-management, and specifically about how the body's nervous system can be tricked by pain sensations. Consider, for example, the familiar pain we call brain freeze.

That's the common experience of feeling a sharp pain in the forehead right between the eyes after you eat or drink something that's icy cold. But when you feel this pain, it simply means that your hypersensitive nervous system is making a mistake. Brain freeze happens if the soft palate at the back of the roof of your mouth detects something really, really cold in there, sending messages to your brain. But your brain can only hint at the general vicinity of where these signals come from. So even though there's absolutely nothing wrong with your forehead, that's where you'll feel brain freeze pain.

Similarly, if you believe you are not getting the right care for your pain, or if there is something dangerous going on around you, you will probably experience more pain than if those external circumstances were not happening.

Taking a pain pill that you believe will work, for instance, can make your sensation of pain start to decrease even before the medication has time to be absorbed into your bloodstream. But what if you open the medicine cabinet in your bathroom and suddenly realize that you've run out of those trusty pain pills? Because your belief now is that you can't get the immediate help you need, your nervous system pays more attention to those pain signals, and you will feel more intense pain.

When it comes to the chest pain of heart attack, even using the word pain to describe this symptom might be inaccurate for some people. Many women do not describe their cardiac chest symptoms as pain at all, for example, instead using words like pressure, aching, burning, heaviness, fullness, or tightness. Some of my blog readers have told me that they actually argued with ER staff who were writing the words "chest pain" on their medical charts: "Well, it's not really 'pain' . . ."

And again, remember that *10 percent of women having a heart attack experience no chest symptoms at all.*[4] None. Nothing. Nada.

Pain in general is nature's way to protect our bodies. Pain has a way of attracting our focused attention in a laser-like fashion, warning us that something might be wrong. For heart patients, there's the initial pain of a cardiac event, and there can also be ongoing pain following treatment for that event. For example, if you've had one or more stents implanted, you may experience what we call "stretching pain" for a while. Although it's common for heart patients to experience some residual pain following a cardiac intervention, such symptoms may sometimes indicate a serious complication—so call your doctor if pain persists or gets worse instead of better over time.

The pain that accompanies a heart attack can be described differently by different people, from "no pain at all" to "worst pain I've ever felt."

Meanwhile, here's my best advice if you or somebody you care about experiences pain or other heart attack symptoms that feel different from anything you've experienced before:

1. *Call 911.* Do not let anybody drive you to the ER. Do not drive yourself.
2. While you're waiting for the ambulance to arrive, chew one regular full-strength (300–500 mg) uncoated aspirin washed down with water—provided that you are not allergic or already taking blood-thinning medications.

How Does It Really Feel to Have a Heart Attack?

Like most women, I'd never really thought much about my heart before my own heart attack—except maybe when running up the killer Quadra Street hill with my running group. Yet heart disease is one of women's biggest health threats each year, killing more women annually than all forms of cancer combined.[5]

Women need to know all of the potential symptoms of a heart attack and seek help if these symptoms do hit. Consider these real-world descriptions shared by female survivors.[6] Some of their stories may surprise you.

S.A., age 37, US: "I woke up at 3 a.m. and my first symptom was heartburn, even though I'd eaten nothing that might cause that. My husband brought me antacids, then a sharp pain went through my back and I told my husband I felt like I was going to die—all in the matter of one minute from the initial symptom. My heart actually stopped and I had to be defibrillated twice in hospital, and then was unconscious for four days. Three more trips to hospital afterwards, but no plaque, just coronary spasms that felt like heartburn, nausea and sometimes chest pain."

Early Warning Signs of a Heart Attack

Several days before I first slumped against that Garry oak on Belmont Avenue, I experienced what doctors call *prodromal symptoms* on two separate occasions in the week leading up to my first trip to the ER. These are early warning signs that something is not quite right. Like most women, I ignored them.

On two days in a row as I walked to work at the hospital, about a thirty-minute brisk walk from home, I had to slow down and then finally stop in front of the same house on Leighton Street just to catch my breath. I was sucking wind like I used to do on that steep Quadra Street hill during long Sunday runs.

This house sits at the top of a slight uphill portion of my walk. I'd been walking up that same little hill day after day for years on my route to work without ever feeling short of breath. But on each of those two days, after I'd waited and rested to see if my symptoms eased up, I didn't give that shortness of breath a second thought for the rest of the day.

When University of Arkansas researcher Dr. Jean McSweeney interviewed hundreds of female heart attack survivors, she discovered something that surprised her: 95 percent of the women she interviewed actually suspected something was wrong in the weeks or months leading up to the heart attacks.[7]

In this research, the most commonly reported early warning prodromal symptoms before a heart attack was finally diagnosed included:

♥ unusual fatigue (71 percent)
♥ sleep disturbance (48 percent)
♥ shortness of breath (42 percent)
♥ chest discomfort (30 percent)

D.W., age 49, US: "I was asleep and woke up not being able to breathe. I felt an ache in my left shoulder blade. My throat felt 'full' and my lips were numb. These symptoms came and went until I ended up in hospital and had four stents implanted. But even before that night, I'd been feeling extremely tired; I kept telling my hubby I wasn't sick, but something was wrong. I never had any chest pain at all until six months after my heart attack."

E.N., age 49, US: "Late one evening, I was working on a website for my son-in-law when I started having some pain in my right arm. I thought that maybe I had worked my arm too much with the computer mouse. But the pain started radiating into my shoulder and after this into my back. There was no pain in my chest. I thought it was time to quit working, and I did some meditation. The next morning, I awoke and felt awful. I could hardly breathe, my back hurt, and I felt like throwing up but could not. The symptoms got steadily worse and I called 911. The firefighters and paramedics who responded knew right away that it was a heart attack when they saw my EKG. When we got to the E.R., however, the doctor told the nurses to take the EKG leads off because I was just having a panic attack. But the paramedics insisted that my leads be placed on again. I was immediately sent by helicopter to a different hospital, where I had three stents implanted. It was very scary."

S.H., age 43, New Zealand: "My heart attack started as I was walking across a flat lawn on my way to feed our goldfish. The pain struck out of the blue. I had no idea that a heart attack could present with pain in the back rather than the chest. My first symptom was a strong pain in between my shoulder blades, a lot like very bad indigestion but in my back instead of my tummy. A few minutes after the pain in my back started, I got very, very hot, and then I felt nauseous. After several minutes, I felt the pain travel through into my centre chest, and then down my left arm to my hand. Like many others, that's when I guessed that this might be serious. The pain kept increasing in my back until it was unbearable, but the other symptoms pretty much stayed the same until I was treated in hospital. Thank heavens for morphine—yay! I was diagnosed with a heart attack, and two stents were implanted. They were tough days."

D.B., age 42, US: "I was under a lot of stress the week I had my heart attack. My first symptom was an odd squeezing sensation in my chest, as if someone reached out and grabbed my heart and squeezed it a few times. No pain—it really didn't hurt. My chest sensations went away after I used my emergency asthma inhaler, as I had mistaken the beginnings of the heart attack as an asthma attack. After my chest sensations eased, my upper back between the shoulder blades started to ache immensely. I felt an odd numbing/tingling sensation move up my arm, which immediately made me worry and was the reason I went to the E.R. as I knew this was a classic heart attack symptom. But my back pain fluctuated, and arm tingling did not go away. In hospital, doctors found a 95% blockage in my left anterior descending coronary artery (LAD–the dreaded 'widow maker' heart attack) that they were going to stent. But after the first stent was implanted, an area in the artery near the stent dissected (tore) and I had to have emergency double bypass open heart surgery. I did not recognize my initial chest sensations and back pain as a heart attack, and as a result I did not seek immediate help. I was subsequently diagnosed with congestive heart failure."

L.D., age 56, UK: "The only symptom of my heart attack was heartburn—first time I'd had heartburn in 26 years since I was pregnant. I had no pain at all, but this heartburn would not go, no matter what I took for it. This was on my birthday, and I'd had too much to eat and drink. I Googled 'heartburn' and up popped 'heart attack symptoms'—so I took an aspirin and went to hospital, where cardiologists implanted a stent in my left anterior descending artery."

L.U., age 40, US: "I was asleep and my symptoms woke me up. I had several simultaneous symptoms, but the first one seemed to be chest pain in the center-left, somewhat under my left breast area. I'd never felt anything like it. It wasn't sharp or crushing or burning, more like a dull pressure. I also had pain down the inside of my left arm that radiated up into the left side of my jaw and my left ear. I was very overheated, and I felt like I was going to throw up. The nausea and overheating faded, but the pain—chest, arm, jaw—stayed. In hospital, I was diagnosed with a heart attack caused by Spontaneous Coronary Artery Dissection (SCAD), treated with six stents."

S.U., age 61, Mauritius: "The sequence of events is so vivid in my mind. Before my heart attack, I had had some shortness of breath after exertion like going upstairs. My first big cardiac symptoms were a discomforting stomach pain and a tightening chest pain that woke me up at 4 a.m. from my sleep. The chest pain gradually radiated down my left arm, a numbing sensation. I started sweating as the pain grew in intensity during my trip to the ER, which took about 25 minutes. I was restless every second, and the pain in my chest became unbearable and tight. These symptoms persisted until I was given an injection and rushed to the Cardiac Unit for angioplasty and one stent implanted in my LAD. As it was placed, all the pain went away."

M.A., age 46, US: "Even before my first obvious symptoms, I had noticed a dead tired, flu-like fatigue, 'tired to the bone through and through,' as I told my son. I almost went home to bed after driving the kids to school (I would be dead now; I needed groceries first though!). I developed heartburn that progressed to a pressure on my chest. I also had a strange aching feeling in my elbows. It was weird, like arthritis that became worse with time. But the most prominent symptom I had, which kept getting stronger and would not go away, was the little voice in my head telling me this was not normal. I wanted to mention this because it is my one piece of advice to

all my friends: 'Listen to that voice in your head!' When we got
to the E.R., they took me right in quickly when staff heard that
I had both chest pain and this odd pain in my elbows. My symptoms did change a bit—one would subside, and another would
get worse. The only one that got much worse was in the elbows.
I had to be airlifted to a hospital with advanced cardiac care.
Cardiologists there found a large unexpected arterial tear diagnosed as Spontaneous Coronary Artery Dissection (SCAD) and
repaired half of it with three stents. They left the other half to heal
itself. Three weeks later, they found that it had indeed healed."

G.L., age 63, Canada: "I had a tremendous, dull, pressing pain
in the centre of my chest, as if a walnut were being pushed into
it. I also had numbness in my right shoulder radiating down my
arm and felt as if the arm suddenly became weighted. Later, the
same symptoms hit in my left shoulder and arm. Chest pain
stayed, but the numbness in both arms gradually went away.
This was replaced with blinding pain in between my shoulder
blades. Once started, the back pain only got worse. I could no
longer sit, stand, lie down or walk around. The pain was so
intense it took my breath away. I remember thinking that these
were signs that you could be having a heart attack. These
events took place between 4 p.m. on Christmas Eve and about
11:30 a.m. on Christmas Day when I finally thought it was
serious enough to get my son to drive me to our local hospital.
These just didn't sound like the classic cardiac symptoms I had
heard of. I lost consciousness while the E.R. doctor was trying
to convince me it was just a gallbladder attack and not a heart
attack. It took three days to stabilize me before I could be flown
to the cardiac hospital in Victoria, where I had an angioplasty
done with two stents implanted. Maybe someone will read this
and decide not to wait as long as I did."

D.I., heart attack at age 33, US: "My first heart attack was
23 years ago but I remember it as though it were yesterday. I
had just turned 33, and had given birth three months before my

heart attack, but even during the pregnancy and afterwards, I had been having chest pains. I'd mentioned it to my ob/gyn, but he told me that they were just pregnancy-related. One night, I put my 3-month old baby to sleep in her crib, checked on my older daughter and went to the living room to relax before heading to bed myself. My first symptom was like a fist in the center of my chest, pushing and squeezing to get out. The pain felt as though someone was gripping me inside right in the center of the sternum and squeezing until I could hardly breathe. My left arm hurt from the shoulder to the elbow, then stopped and picked up hurting at my wrist into my hand. I started feeling very sick to my stomach and vomited until there was nothing left, but still continued retching. I was sweating like crazy. I woke up my husband, and told him I thought I was having a heart attack, but not really believing that! While waiting for the ambulance, I went from abnormal sweating to freezing cold. In hospital, they diagnosed a 98% blockage of the LAD. I spent 15 days in hospital. My second heart attack happened 10 years ago when I was 46. I was having ongoing problems with unstable angina so I had to have a stent implanted. The day after I came home from hospital, I walked into my living room and all of a sudden, I had this overwhelming feeling that something was terribly wrong. I told my husband to call 911. In hospital, they stabilized me and sent me to another hospital, where a cardiologist attempted to open up the new stent that had just been implanted. It had closed up, causing another heart attack. I went into cardiac arrest twice. I am now 56 and in need of bypass surgery for another blockage in the circumflex artery which they are unable to stent."

K.A., age 55, US: "I awoke around 1:30 a.m. and felt pain down my right arm. It intensified as time went on, with the pain/tightness extending to my chest area. I had intense nausea and began vomiting and having bouts of horrible diarrhea in between. When I got to the hospital, the cardiologist found my

LAD had collapsed without any coronary artery disease. While he was implanting two stents, he caused a hole in my artery, so had to put in a third stent. Even before that night, I'd felt flu-ish with no energy, but didn't think that was unusual because I also live with Chronic Fatigue Syndrome."

M.O., heart attack at age 32, US: "For one month prior to my heart attack, I was not feeling well with chest pains, lockjaw and fatigue. But my first real symptom began at 5 a.m.—pain in mid-chest radiating into my back and up into my throat. I felt like I was being strangled, pain spreading into my throat and ears. The pain literally felt like 10,000 elephants sitting on my chest. In the ER, because of my young age and the fact that I weighed only 100 pounds soaking wet, they thought I was a drug user. I was later told I'd had a massive heart attack. I spent two days being stabilized before having a stent implanted, but instead of the stent, I was taken straight in for emergency bypass surgery. My heart now has severe damage to the lower left chamber. Last spring, 10 years after my heart attack, I had to go back into hospital to have an implantable cardioverter defibrillator (ICD) put into my chest. I have named my ICD 'Trigger'!"

A.L., age 51, US: "I've had two serious cardiac events with different symptoms for each one. My first symptom in January was incredible fatigue. I was sitting in bed, watching TV and could suddenly no longer even hold my head up. The next day began six weeks of on-and-off symptoms of nausea, dizziness, back pain in my left shoulder blade like a muscle knot (which eventually began to radiate through to my chest), profuse night sweats and feelings of being intolerably hot. I began having panic attacks (my first ever), feelings of doom, and severe anxiety. My symptoms were not related to exertion. When I went to the hospital, I had to have emergency open heart surgery for a triple bypass. But almost immediately after my surgery, the bypass grafts began to fail. My chest pain this time felt sharp and pinching as if my clothes were too tight, then it moved up the left side of my neck. My throat felt full, and it was hard to swallow. My left jaw ached (like a dull toothache, or maybe like having a piece of popcorn stuck). These symptoms came and went for over two months and were ignored by my cardiologist because he said they were different than my pre-bypass symptoms. Finally, I was correctly diagnosed and had two stents implanted to open the failed bypass grafts."

M.Y., age 26, US: "I was 35 weeks pregnant and feeling really tired because we had just put up the new baby crib the night before. I went to sleep, but woke up to this weird constricting feeling in my lower throat, like I had a lump of something stuck there. The feeling went down to my upper chest and continued down to the lower chest area. It was not pain, just more of a squeezing, restricting feeling. I then started to get a slight pain that felt like acid reflux. I started to feel faint so I woke up my husband. I was sweating profusely, nauseated, had the chills and felt faint. And I also had a very weird tingling and numbness in BOTH arms from my shoulders to my elbows. We went to the hospital, where I was told that I'd had a massive heart attack caused by an aneurysm. It had exploded and made a tear in one of my heart valves, allowing blood to flow through the layers and squeeze the valve. The doctors said my body just couldn't handle the stress of the pregnancy. I ended up having an emergency C-section and triple bypass surgery. I have also had an ICD implanted because my heart muscle has not healed. But even before that day, I'd been feeling tired and short of breath, and I had just blamed it on being pregnant. Now I can see all these issues as cardiac problems and not just pregnancy."

J.O., age 60, US: "I had experienced some symptoms in the weeks before my heart attack, such as tightness in the chest and extreme pain in my left shoulder blade. I also had these same symptoms months earlier, but dismissed them as just a pulled muscle after lifting heavy luggage. My doctor thought I had pleurisy or a virus but he sent my EKG (with an unusual

T-wave) to the cardiologist who wanted me to come in for the stress test. My heart attack actually happened on the stress treadmill in the cardiologist's office! I had extreme shortness of breath but felt no pain. He handed me a nitroglycerin tablet to put under my tongue. I was lucky to have my heart attack on the treadmill, because a subsequent angiogram showed no blockages, but a spasm diagnosis of Prinzmetal's Angina."

K.M., age 52, US: "I'd been feeling extremely tired for some time. One day, I was putting the vacuum cleaner away, and suddenly felt as if I'd pulled a muscle in my chest, in the center of my sternum, like a tight, heavy pain. I was sweating pro-fusely and feeling nauseated. I had pain/tingling in my left arm, and then I blacked out. When the paramedics arrived, they gave me nitroglycerin which eased the symptoms temporarily. In hospital, I had to have two stents implanted and spent two days in ICU because of low blood pressure."

A.M., heart attack at age 28, US: "I had crushing chest pain while I was pregnant, along with sweating and nausea, but I was told it was just the baby kicking my diaphragm. These symptoms continued for two years, off and on, usually brought on by exertion. After pregnancy, I was told it was just exercise-induced asthma, then pleurisy. Finally, after a bad episode (burning up and down my chest—like heartburn on steroids, sweating, nausea, vomiting, tingling in my arms and legs—both sides, stabbing shoulder pain and shortness of breath), I was finally sent for a treadmill stress test. By this time, even walking across the room or watching something emotional on TV (like a Hallmark card commercial!) would set off symptoms. I was taken to hospital, but during my angiogram, I had a massive heart attack on the table. I had to be transferred to another hospital and had emergency double bypass surgery. Since that first heart attack, I've had a second heart attack and double bypass surgery at age 30, nine cardiac stents and three iliac artery stents implanted at 30 and 31, and then triple bypass surgery at age 31."

K.R., age 46, US: "My first heart attack was on May 7, and my second was on May 22. My first symptoms felt like a blow to the chest, like a shotgun smack dab in the middle of my chest. It immediately took my breath away and knocked me backwards about 3–4 feet. I also had an intense drilling pain under my left funny bone. The symptoms did not let up. At the time, I was just sitting at my desk. Doctors found 0% plaque in my arteries—I was diagnosed with a coronary artery spasm from Prinzmetal's Variant Angina. I remained several days at two different hospitals."

G.L., age 49, UK: "I had what I later found out was classic angina, severe tiredness and increasing chest pain, misdiagnosed and treated for all sorts of things, including inflammation of the sternum, but it got steadily worse over six months. I then had an angiogram that showed severe disease in two of my coronary arteries. I was treated with various medications over six months, but steadily worsened. Then doctors attempted a stent placement that failed, and I was sent home the same day with a small dissection (tear) which I was told would heal by itself. But two days after the dissection, I had increasingly unstable angina unresponsive to nitroglycerin, with sweating and nausea. I went to the E.R. where I had a bigger heart attack, with crushing pain, pain radiating up into my throat and tongue, nausea, vomiting and sweating, plus pain in my left arm. These symptoms came and went, in between different drugs they were giving me. A further angiogram showed that the dissection had not healed but extended, and the artery was full of blood clots. I was then sent immediately by ambulance with police escort to a cardiac unit a couple of counties away, where I had four stents implanted. This did not cure the problem, however, so two months ago I had to have double bypass open heart surgery."

2 ♡ Deadly Delay

By the time I return home from my morning walk (following that little detour at Emergency), I'm feeling pretty normal, albeit very embarrassed for having made such a big deal out of a simple case of heartburn.

But I don't have to wait long before something else happens.

The next afternoon, I'm sitting in my office at the hospice, noodling away at the computer, just one building over from the one housing our hospital's Emergency Department that I'd visited yesterday. Although it's only springtime, I'm already starting on my next big public relations project: our non-profit society's annual report that I'll be distributing at our annual general meeting in the fall.

Suddenly, out of nowhere, I'm blindsided by a repeat of the exact symptoms that had forced me to stop my walk the day before. Central chest pain. Nausea. Sweating. That damned pain down my left arm.

But unlike the last time they struck, I now know from what that ER physician told me that these symptoms are not heart-related. What I also know is that all I have to do is wait about 15 or 20 minutes, and these symptoms will likely fade, just like they did yesterday.

And so that's what I do, leaning over my keyboard, puffing Lamaze breaths through the pain and the nausea and the cold sweat that's threatening my new white cotton blouse. Sure enough, as expected, the symptoms seem to ease up after several minutes.

Identical symptoms strike again the next day at work, and then again on the day after that, and the day after that. I am amazed at how awful heartburn feels. How can people stand this? By the end of the week, I'm popping Gaviscon like candy. But I certainly have no intention of embarrassing myself again by returning to the ER. And I do have an appointment to discuss this acid reflux with my longtime family doctor as soon as she gets back from her vacation.

After almost two weeks of increasingly frequent acid reflux symptoms, I board a plane and fly to Ottawa to help celebrate my mother's eightieth birthday.

By now, I'm becoming pretty good at learning to somehow normalize these daily episodes, and even better at hiding them from a large extended family of my brothers, sisters, assorted nieces, nephews, in-laws, and many other relatives and close friends—but especially from my mom. This is her special weekend, and many people have flown in from all across the country just to celebrate her life. Despite my worsening symptoms, I don't want to make any kind of fuss that could ruin her party. A three-generation photo taken that weekend of my mother, my daughter, Larissa, and me shows my best public relations smiley-face. I'm fine, just fine. . . .

When they strike, the worst chest pain episodes feel like a cross between a Mack truck parked on my chest and a fiery deep burn roaring right up into my throat. The episodes become much worse by the end of the weekend when my son, Ben, drops me off at the Ottawa airport to fly home: two severe attacks at the airport, and two even worse ones during that five-hour late-night flight to Vancouver.

At no time do I consider calling the flight attendant over to ask for help. Although I suspect that something might be very wrong, I don't want to become one of those passengers they have to turn the plane around for due to a medical emergency. And really, how embarrassing would that be—all for a case of acid reflux?

All I can think about is that soon, I will be home, and everything will somehow be okay.

When the plane finally lands in Vancouver, I'm faced with a dilemma. I'm feeling so ill by now that I can barely walk five steps, but I need to get to my next gate to catch the 25-minute connector flight to my island home here in Victoria.

So I flag down a passing Air Canada golf cart, and hitch a ride to the far end of Vancouver's airport. Once onboard my connector flight, I can already see another problem looming. I realize that when we land, I won't be able to walk from the plane to the Victoria airport baggage carousel for my suitcases. And that's when I finally decide to call a flight attendant over. "Could you please arrange for a wheelchair to meet me when we land in Victoria?"

She smiles, and asks if I'm okay.

"I'm fine. I'm just having trouble walking."

(This, by the way, is absolutely true. I am having trouble walking. A lot of trouble.)

When the plane lands in Victoria, the wheelchair awaits. A few minutes later, I somehow manage to heave two suitcases onto a luggage cart and head out to the airport's long-term parking lot, where, yes, I get behind the wheel of my little green car. But the exertion of getting my bags loaded leaves me shaky and weak, and honestly, I just don't know how on earth I'm going to drive.

Denial during a Cardiac Crisis

What I've just described during that two-week nightmare now seems like a case of denial on steroids. How could I possibly have interpreted my symptoms as simple heartburn, even as they worsened day by day? I'm not a physician, but even I knew that pain down your left arm isn't a sign of acid reflux, so why did I continue to cling so dangerously to what that ER doctor had told me? My account of what happened in that airport parking lot continues in the next chapter, but meanwhile, here's a famously true story popular among those who study the intriguing phenomenon of denial during a crisis.

It's about the 1987 King's Cross subway fire in London. As unbelievable as it may seem, and even as the fire in the underground tube station continued to spread, trains kept on arriving in the station, and hurrying evening commuters headed right into the disaster. Some officials unwittingly directed passengers onto escalators that carried them straight into the fire below. Many commuters followed their regular routines despite the greasy black smoke churning out of the entrances, seemingly oblivious to the crush of people trying to escape—some of them actually in flames. At least three employees were notified by passengers of smoke and flames, yet none of the three called the fire department. Over 30 people perished in the tragic King's Cross fire.

It turns out that social scientists have another name for this mystifying phenomenon: the *incredulity response*. As described by UK survival psychologist Dr. John Leach in an interview with *Newsweek*,[1] people experiencing a crisis like the King's Cross fire may simply not believe what they're seeing with their own eyes, so they go about their business, engaging in what's known as *normalcy bias*. They may act as if everything is fine, while significantly underestimating the seriousness of their circumstances. You're probably familiar with normalcy bias if you've ever automatically assumed that the clanging fire alarm doesn't actually mean fire. Normalcy bias is incredibly powerful, and sometimes downright hazardous.

It neatly sums up how I responded while undergoing those two weeks of increasingly debilitating symptoms. Although all signs clearly pointed to a potential heart attack, I seemed fatalistically determined to go about my life behaving as if all around me was fine, just fine.

But we're in a bit of a time crunch when in the middle of a heart attack. That critically important period of time between first symptoms and actively getting the help we need to open up (or revascularize) blocked coronary arteries can be divided into three basic phases:

1. *decision time*—the period from the first onset of acute cardiac symptoms to the decision to seek care (for example, calling 911)
2. *transport time*—the period from the decision to seek care to the arrival at the ER
3. *therapy time*—the period from arrival at Emergency to the start of appropriate medical treatment

Only the first phase is the one you have complete control over. So don't blow it.

Part of the reason for my own freakishly dangerous treatment-seeking delay decision was that misinformed stereotype I held about the type of person who suffers a heart attack (i.e., not a person like me). Very few of us believe we look like that person. As a former distance runner, I never imagined that I was even remotely at risk. And what did turn out to be one of my most significant cardiac risk factors (a history of serious pregnancy complications) wasn't even on my radar until two years after I survived that heart attack. I was pitifully ignorant about heart disease before surviving my own cardiac event.

And besides, I was also still able to walk, talk, remain conscious, make decisions, drive, go to work, fly to Ottawa for my mother's birthday weekend (all signs of normalcy), while suffering increasingly debilitating cardiac symptoms. No wonder I was in full-blown denial.

Dr. Leach has a well-known theory about how experiences like mine, indicating a seemingly bizarre disregard for an obvious health threat, can so often occur.[2] During a crisis, for example, most of us will quite simply feel stunned and bewildered. We may find that our reasoning is significantly impaired and that thinking is difficult. We'll behave in a reflexive, almost automatic, or mechanical manner. We may experience perceptual narrowing or tunnel vision. And the more upset we become, the more our decision-making skills can be affected.

Refusing to acknowledge that something's wrong can be a common way of coping with a serious health crisis, emotional conflict, threatening information, intense stress, painful thoughts, or anxiety—especially at the beginning. We remain in denial about what makes us feel vulnerable or threatens our sense of control. Such denial can serve as a remarkably effective defense mechanism, useful to help reduce anxiety by trying to reduce that perceived threat—but not when we're in mid–heart attack.

Would You Rather Be Embarrassed—or Dead?

Looking back, I can see how foolish it must seem to admit that I felt too embarrassed to go back for emergency medical help as soon as those distressing cardiac symptoms returned. Too embarrassed to let family members and friends at my mother's birthday party know that I was in trouble. Too embarrassed to ask the flight attendants for help during that endless flight home from Ottawa, or to refuse to board that flight in the first place.

But Len Gould understands this embarrassment well. He's an Australian psychologist who runs a cardiac rehabilitation program for heart patients—but more importantly to me, he's also a heart patient himself

Women's Treatment-Seeking Delay Behavior

I have long thought that the most dramatic part of my story was not that my heart attack had been misdiagnosed, but that for some insane reason, I refused to go back to Emergency until I could no longer bear my symptoms. Denial? Embarrassment? Stupidity?

It turns out that this reaction among female heart patients is so common that researchers actually study what they call treatment-seeking delay behavior. One such research team was led by Dr. Anne Rosenfeld of Oregon Health and Science University's School of Nursing.[3] The team identified six important patterns of treatment-seeking delay behavior in female heart attack survivors. They called these patterns:

- ♥ *Knowing and going* (women acknowledged something was wrong, made a decision to seek care, and acted on their decision within a relatively short time, typically 5–15 minutes).
- ♥ *Knowing and letting someone else take over* (women told someone they had symptoms and were willing to go along with recommendations to seek immediate medical care).
- ♥ *Knowing and going on the patient's own terms* (women wanted to remain in control, were not willing to let others make decisions for them, and openly acknowledged that they did not like to ask others for help; these are the women who often drive themselves to Emergency).
- ♥ *Knowing and waiting* (women decided that they needed help, but delayed seeking treatment because they did not want to disturb others).
- ♥ *Managing an alternative hypothesis* (women decided symptoms were due to indigestion or other non-cardiac causes, and were reluctant to call 911 "in case there's nothing wrong and I'd feel like a fool"—until their severe symptoms changed or became unbearable).
- ♥ *Minimizing* (women tried to ignore their symptoms or hoped the symptoms would go away, and did not recognize that their symptoms were heart-related).

The common lesson running throughout each of many studies on women's treatment-seeking delay decisions during a heart attack is this:

You know your body.

You know when something is just not right.

Call 911 right away if you start experiencing troubling symptoms that you suspect are heart-related—in other words, as soon as you identify that these symptoms do not feel normal for you.

who has undergone coronary artery bypass surgery. He recently emailed me about this disturbingly pervasive tendency toward being embarrassed to seek medical help even when we're experiencing obvious cardiac symptoms. He shared two typical examples of how pervasive—and potentially dangerous—this embarrassment can be:

Last night, at one of my cardiac rehab sessions, a group member told me that he had not called the ambulance when he had a heart attack at work because he did not want to be embarrassed in front of his workmates.

And many partners or friends can make it worse when they make fun of people who call for help if it's finally determined that the symptoms were not heart-related.

Another example: a colleague of mine recently had chest pain and went to the local Emergency ward (as he should). However, a number of people have since told this story as "Bill's little attention-seeking episode." Naturally, this will impact any future decisions Bill makes about seeking medical help or not.[4]

My own best advice for Bill (and for anybody else who's feeling reluctant to seek emergency help when experiencing cardiac symptoms that just don't feel right) is based on Len's wise words: "Don't be embarrassed to death."

Denial after a Cardiac Crisis

Patients already diagnosed, treated, and recovering from a cardiac event can also be in a state of denial, even while still in the hospital. For example, we may say things like:

"I just can't believe this."
"This couldn't be happening to me."
"Well, doctors do make mistakes!"

What can you do if you too are already diagnosed, but still in denial?

1. Research! Research! Research! Find out as much as you can from credible sources about your diagnosis. When you search online, remember that you need to be a smart consumer in order to tell the difference between the trash and the truth out there. Health information found on university, government, hospital, or non-profit organization websites is generally more reliable than information on websites lacking scientific references or trying to sell you something. Check the resources section at the back of this book for a list of good places to start your research.
2. Listen to medical advice for help in decision making.
3. Listen to your body (pay attention to any distressing signs and symptoms, especially if they worsen or don't feel normal to you).
4. Listen to your health care professionals. Medical professionals can repeat the clinical facts to you, but it's up to you to believe them.

In Denial—Even Around Our Doctors

Leslea Steffel-Dennis is, like me, a graduate of the WomenHeart Science and Leadership training program at Mayo Clinic. She's a heart disease survivor who co-facilitates the WomenHeart support community meetings for women living with heart disease in Thurston County, Washington—one of over 100 such groups across the US and Canada.[5]

Leslea wrote to me about a surprisingly common type of denial seen in already-diagnosed female heart patients, and specifically about this question: How good should we look for our doctor's appointment?[6] When we're heading out the door for these appointments, should we let our doctors see reality, or should they see only our best smiley-face pretense that we are *"Fine, just fine"*—even when we're not fine at all? Leslea described her own tendencies like this:

> Having nails nicely polished hot red, so the doc can't see any symptom that would show up in my fingernails.
>
> Or a thick slather of foundation to hide the sick color my skin really is. And don't forget to put some on the bruise marks from the heart meds.
>
> And when the Doc asks how you feel, it's not the time to say, "Well, I felt a whole lot worse when I made the appointment, but I'm pretty good now!"

In other words, don't make a fuss. Don't draw attention to yourself. It's not that bad. Don't whine. Don't complain. Just get on with it. Smile sweetly and try to act normal.

Leslea's list also brings up the maddeningly typical tendency of so many of us to try to minimize or dismiss cardiac symptoms in general, while clinging to that concept of normalcy bias that Dr. Leach shares. But while a temporary denial of reality may serve as a type of natural coping mechanism that gives us a bit more time to adjust, little by little, to a painful reality that feels almost too big to comprehend, prolonged denial can become a problem. Staying in denial can interfere with both effective solutions and our ability to follow basic medical instructions, affecting the way we're able to face challenges that lie ahead. Denying a current reality can also lead to postponing the inevitable when that reality finally comes crashing down on us.

Most importantly, never keep the truth about how you're feeling a secret from your own physician. Even the most skilled and caring medical team can't help you if the team doesn't know the truth about what you're going through. Maybe, as Leslea now recommends, we could skip the nail polish, the foundation, and the stoic determination to look good on the outside in order to mask the reality inside. Maybe the doctor's notes in our charts will start reflecting reality instead of the fiction we help to spread by pretending to be "fine, just fine."

Where Are You on Your Own Priority List?

While attending the WomenHeart Science and Leadership training at Mayo Clinic, I heard the prominent cardiologist Dr. Sharonne Hayes (founder of the Mayo Women's Heart Clinic and director of their Office of Diversity and Inclusion) report on a survey conducted earlier at Mayo.[7] The survey asked female participants this one question:

"What is most important to you in life?"

Whenever I do presentations about women's heart health now, I like to ask my audiences to guess in advance the correct order of this study's top six answers, just for fun. These rankings are surprising, in an amusing-yet-oddly-pathetic way. The order of our reported priorities may also help to explain why, even when some women are experiencing deadly heart attack symptoms, they will delay seeking treatment if something more important crops up.

More important? What could possibly be more important when you're having a heart attack? But when asked to prioritize their lives, women who were surveyed ranked priorities like this:

1. *Children:* Our local newspaper ran a story recently of a mother who threw herself between her toddler and the wild cougar who had attacked the child during a hike in the woods. Think about this. How many times, as a new mom, when you were feeling desperately ill, at death's door, puking and feverish, did you drag yourself out of your sickbed in order to feed the baby or drive the kids to hockey practice? Who else on earth would you do this for? I blame motherhood for a lot of my selflessness.

2. *Home:* Women care a lot about our homes, big or small. Feeling responsible for providing a clean, comfortable, safe, and attractive family home is near the top of our priority lists. And let's face it, if your house is a complete pigsty because you just haven't had the time or energy to clean, your visitors will never say, "Boy, is he a messy housekeeper!"

3. *Work:* Whether we have children at home or not, women rate their careers in the middle of our priority lists. How we spend our hours in the workplace is important to us in ways that go beyond just a paycheck, from social relationships with co-workers to intellectual stimulation and increased self-esteem.

4. *Pets:* This priority listing always draws a knowing laugh from my women's heart health presentation audiences. We do love our pets! When Canadian researchers studied the psychosocial benefits of pet ownership, they reported that the unconditional love inherent in having a pet increased owners' feelings of belonging, self-esteem, and meaningful existence, and even motivated healthy behaviors.[8]

5. *Spouse:* Significant others are of course on this list. Just below the dog. While this result may seem odd and even shocking at first (we love the dog more than the spouse?), see #4 for possible explanations for this ranking order.

6. *Myself:* Here's the pathetic part. Women invariably put themselves last on this list. Women from birth are socialized to be nurturers and caretakers of both family and friends, sometimes even at the expense of our own health.[9] In fact, when we do take time for ourselves, we can often feel like we're being selfish, which, as we all know, is the worst possible way to be. And we may actually resent others who spend time on themselves. By comparison, we're relentlessly applauded for selfless sacrifice: "How does Mary do it? She does so much on so little sleep!"

It took a heart attack for me to finally admit that I actually need to put my own health needs first, trusting that the Earth will somehow continue to spin on its axis even if I'm not running everything myself.

If you find yourself experiencing frightening symptoms you believe might be heart related, ask yourself what you'd do if these symptoms were happening to your daughter, your mother, your sister, or any other woman you care about. Chances are you'd insist on seeking immediate help for them.

Why won't we do the same for ourselves?

3 ♡ Finally, a Correct Diagnosis

It's now almost 1:30 in the morning. It takes me a full 20 minutes, sitting in the dark behind the wheel of my little green car in the airport parking lot, before I can decide if I'm capable of driving myself home after the latest assault of symptoms.

This is the worst I've ever felt. I'm shaky, sweaty, sick, and exhausted. If I could only somehow manage to get myself home . . .

I put the car into gear and start rolling, as if testing my ability to remember how this driving thing works. I stop at the parking attendant's booth. I say nothing to the young man inside as I fumble with the cash I've pulled from my wallet, willing my brain to connect the synapses between the weekend parking fee he requests with the bills in my hand. I try to smile as he hands me my change, bids me good night, and watches as I drive off. Luckily, at this time of night, there's virtually no traffic on the roads as I leave the airport. I manage to make it home and park the car.

By now, I'm focused only on moving slowly. I unlock the door and crash into bed, fully clothed, boots still on, and wait for morning to arrive. I've already decided to return to Emergency, but not now, of course. No, I'll go in the morning, right after shift change, when the staff are fresh, which my foggy brain decides is the optimal time to go to the ER. I just need to get some powerful drugs to treat this acid reflux.

When the sun rises and I do show up in the ER, I can tell right away simply by the looks on the faces of the staff that something is very different from the last time I was here two weeks ago. I strain to understand the buzz of urgent whispers I hear outside my curtained cubicle. This time, a cardiologist is called in (which didn't happen two weeks earlier).

He is an extremely tall man wearing some kind of crazy Hawaiian-print shirt and truly impressive shoulder-length black hair. I catch a glimpse of him from my gurney, and wonder if he is the cardiologist I've been told is on the way. I recall thinking that most women would kill to have shiny spiral curls like his. He doesn't look like any physician I've ever met—and I've worked in this hospital for many years. He approaches my bedside and introduces himself to me, gently taking my hand with both of his own.

"Mrs. Thomas, I can tell from looking at all of your tests, and your T-waves, that you have significant heart disease."

Significant heart disease.

Significant heart disease?

Did he just say "significant heart disease"?

From that moment on, although I can hear more words coming out of his mouth, and I can see his lips moving, he might as well be speaking Swahili. I simply cannot comprehend what's being said. I suspect he might be talking about what happens next if a person has significant heart disease. I may have signed a piece of paper that I'm guessing now was a consent form. When I catch words that sound like medical procedures, I raise one hand to interrupt. I ask him if I should make an appointment while I'm here to book these procedures for another day.

He smiles at me and shakes his head. "No. We're taking you straight upstairs. Right now." I don't know it at the time, but I'm soon to learn that the question I'd just asked is remarkably common among freshly diagnosed and confused heart patients.

More foreign words, and then the words *heart attack*.

I interrupt again: "Wait. Are you saying that I'm going to have a heart attack?"

"No. I'm saying that you are having a heart attack."

More sounds, more lips moving. None of it makes sense.

A hospital porter arrives to take me immediately upstairs to the cardiac unit. As my gurney is hurried down the corridor, a woman passes who does a quick double take when she sees my face, and then starts jogging alongside me as we head toward the elevator.

"Carolyn?" I look up and recognize the mother of one of Ben's school friends. I haven't seen Andrea for years. Looking concerned, she asks, "What's happening? What are you doing here?"

And that's when I feel my eyes stinging and hot tears starting down both cheeks.

"They say I'm having a heart attack."

How Does a Cardiac Misdiagnosis Happen?

There is still, amazingly, a persistent myth that heart disease is a man's disease. Even the name of the type of heart attack I survived (the so-called widow maker) tells you a lot. The words reflect the historical assumption that this kind of heart attack affects men, not women. Doctors don't, after all, call it the widower maker.

Some in the medical profession may still be reluctant to consider heart disease, even when a woman presents with the same obvious cardiac symptoms I had. An American Heart Association survey of physicians showed that only 8 percent of family physicians (and worse, 17 percent of cardiologists) were aware that heart disease kills more women than men each year, a statistic that's been true since 1984.[1]

Women with heart disease are far more likely than men to be misdiagnosed. Research on cardiac misdiagnoses reported in the *New England Journal of Medicine* suggested that women in their fifties or younger were seven times more likely to be misdiagnosed during a heart attack than their male counterparts.[2] The consequences of this were significant: being sent away from the hospital doubled the risk of dying.

We also know that physicians are more likely to assess a woman's cardiac symptoms as being psychological instead of heart-related. A landmark Cardiovascular Research Foundation study, for example, found that when doctors reviewed case studies of both men and women who had presented to Emergency with classic heart attack symptoms, along with a recent history of an emotionally upsetting personal event, they were significantly more likely to recommend referral of the male patients for further cardiac testing compared to the female patients, who were more likely to have their symptoms dismissed as being due simply to the recent emotional upset.[3]

Researchers found that just the mention of emotional upset shifted the interpretation of women's chest pain and other cardiac symptoms so that these were thought to have a psychological origin. By contrast, men's identical symptoms were interpreted as heart-related whether or not emotional stressors were present. The results showed a significant gender bias when cardiac symptoms occurred in the context of stress. For example:

♥ vastly fewer women received coronary heart disease diagnoses compared to men (15 percent versus 56 percent)

♥ far fewer women were referred to a cardiologist (30 percent versus 62 percent)

♥ remarkably fewer women were prescribed standard cardiac medications (13 percent versus 47 percent)

I now believe that there are very few experiences in life more anxiety-producing than fearing you might actually be having a heart attack. Unless you arrive at Emergency unconscious, in fact, my guess is that most of you would look and sound highly anxious while in the throes of a cardiac event.

How to Help Yourself Get an Accurate Medical Diagnosis

♥ Know your facts (make notes about when symptoms hit, how often, how severe, and what makes them feel worse/better)

♥ Be specific (stick to your story)

♥ Be thorough (don't leave out the important stuff)

What to do if you think you've been misdiagnosed:

♥ Do not feel embarrassed to speak up and ask clarifying questions such as "What else could this be?"

♥ Ask if there are other or repeat tests possible

♥ Request a second opinion

♥ Keep going back, or go to another medical facility, until you are diagnosed appropriately

♥ Do not lose hope

So if you're a woman, you might be alarmed to learn that this study's results suggest that if you exhibit signs of anxiety, your heart attack symptoms are more likely to be misinterpreted compared to those of men presenting with the same symptoms. And then, on top of your physically distressing cardiac symptoms, you'll also be suffering profound embarrassment and shame over making a fuss about nothing.

Surely, you might be saying to yourself by now, women's cardiac care has improved since these studies were published. But we need only consider the American Heart Association (AHA)'s scientific statement on women and heart attacks released in January, 2016. I would describe the statement's overall conclusion like this:

"Sucks to be female. Better luck next life!"[4]

Of course, you won't actually spot this succinct summary within the pages of the statement, but that's basically the message. That pithy summary, by the way, comes originally from Laura Haywood-Cory, who at age 40 survived a heart attack caused by spontaneous coronary artery dissection.[5]

I haven't decided what upset me most about this AHA scientific statement. Was it the document's conclusion that *heart disease in women remains underdiagnosed and undertreated* compared to our male counterparts? Or was it the fact that it was, shockingly, the first-ever scientific statement on heart attacks in women that the Association has produced in its entire 92-year history?

The AHA statement also reports that tools physicians depend on to help guide them toward an appropriate diagnosis can play a role in this gender gap in cardiac care. Women are less likely than men to receive some diagnostic tests in the first place, and some tests don't work as well in women. Most standard tests for diagnosing heart disease, for example, have been fine-tuned in studies focused for decades on (white, middle-aged) men.

Mayo Clinic cardiologist Dr. Sharonne Hayes offers this informed take on issues surrounding cardiac diagnostic tests in women:

Misconceptions about women's heart disease grew roots decades ago. In the 1960s, erroneous assertions that heart disease was a man's disease were widely spread to the medical community and to the public. This led to research on diagnostics and treatment almost exclusively focused on cardiovascular disease in men.

Many clinical trials and research studies in the past excluded women, or simply didn't make an effort to enroll women in sufficient numbers to draw sex-based conclusions.[6]

Dr. Hayes also believes that misdiagnosis in women may be due to existing cardiac treatment protocols being ignored. "Guidelines can help women get the care that has been shown to improve survival and long term outcomes in large groups of patients. Part of the problem now is that these guidelines are less likely to be applied to women compared to men. We know that when hospitals have systems in place to ensure they provide care according to the guidelines, women's cardiac outcomes improve, even more than men's."

I've come to the sad conclusion that successfully navigating the gatekeepers working in Emergency Medicine (and thus being appropriately diagnosed and referred immediately for treatment) may indeed be the most treacherous part of surviving a cardiac event, especially for women. Once diagnostic test results are identified as normal, as mine were, you suddenly have a new problem: most if not all physicians will quickly move on to consider non-cardiac alternative causes, no matter how alarming your cardiac symptoms might be.

Throw in atypical cardiac symptoms that are more frequently seen in women compared to men, and you may never see an order for those diagnostic tests in the first place. And remember that *at least 10 percent of women experience no chest symptoms of any kind during a heart attack.*[7] This means no chest pain, no pressure, no aching, no fullness, no heaviness, no burning. Nothing.

For both women and men, the decision to seek emergency help in the first place means that symptoms are by definition distressing enough to warrant this action. And although chest pain is the most frequent heart attack symptom reported in both male and female heart attack patients, just imagine being dismissed because you're a woman having a heart attack who, like 10 percent of your sisterhood, fails to demonstrate any chest pain at all.

Here's an example of how an appropriate cardiac diagnosis could look in real life. A woman attending one of my heart health presentations told me of her recent trip to the ER of our local hospital, and an overheard conversation between the doctor and the (male) patient lying in the bed next to her beyond the curtain: "Your blood tests came back fine, your EKG tests are fine, but we're going to admit you for observation just to rule out a heart attack."

How I wish I could have heard those words during my first trip to Emergency. I now believe that if only that ER physician had simply Googled my symptoms (central chest pain, nausea, sweating, and pain down my left arm), both he and Dr. Google would have come up with only one plausible diagnosis: *myocardial infarction* (heart attack).

In that overheard ER conversation, a male patient is thus admitted to a cardiac observation unit in the hospital because of troubling symptoms, even with normal cardiac test results—just as current treatment guidelines recommend.[8] But I and other women in mid–heart attack are being sent home from Emergency following normal test results like his, with misdiagnoses ranging from indigestion to anxiety, stress, gall bladder problems, or menopause (a handy all-purpose misdiagnosis).

Male-Pattern versus Female-Pattern Heart Disease

Why are many women still being underdiagnosed and undertreated compared to male heart patients? Los Angeles cardiologist Dr. Noel Bairey Merz recommends a memorably creative way to address this question. She sums up our basic heart attack differences like this:

"Men explode, but women erode."[9]

She describes the classic Hollywood heart attack accompanied by horrible chest pain, caused by a large blockage that ruptures and explodes within a coronary artery. It's easier for physicians to suspect this kind of massive lesion on diagnostic tests like a clearly abnormal EKG or blood enzyme test. She calls this kind of cardiac event the *male-pattern heart attack*. This pattern does not necessarily occur for women, however. She explains: "Some women have those heart attacks, too, but many have another kind of heart attack where plaque erodes. It may not completely fill the coronary artery with a big clot, the symptoms can be more subtle, her EKG findings are different. That's a *female-pattern heart attack.*"

This approach suggests that the type of fatty plaque seen in the coronary arteries of some women may be deposited differently than in men. Dr. Bairey Merz and her colleagues at Cedars-Sinai Women's Heart Center have observed that the big coronary artery blockage in a man having a heart attack resembles what she calls "a beer belly in his coronary artery," unlike the plaque in women's arteries, which she describes as "very smooth, just laid down nice and tidy."

These differences have only recently been identified, largely because, as Dr. Sharonne Hayes mentioned, for decades most cardiology research has been done on (white, middle-aged) males.[10] So if women's heart disease wasn't being studied, sex-specific results weren't being published in medical journals or discussed at medical meetings. This is why advances in bridging this gender gap in cardiology have happened mostly in recent history. It was only in 2004, for example, that the first recommendations on managing cardiovascular risk factors for women were published in the heart journal *Circulation.*[11]

It makes sense to keep in mind that, as cardiologist Dr. Nieca Goldberg summed up in the catchy title of her book on women's heart health, *Women Are Not Small Men.*[12] Are cardiac diagnostic tools that are designed, researched, and tested mostly on men as accurate in diagnosing women? Are cardiac procedures that are designed, researched, and tested mostly on men as effective in treating women? Are cardiac drugs that are designed, researched, and tested mostly on men as safe or as effective when put into women's bodies?

As if human research that excluded women wasn't bad enough, it turns out that, astonishingly, even the laboratory animals used in most cardiac drug and treatment research until 2014 shared one trait: they were almost exclusively male. Scientists didn't like to use female mice, rats, or pigs in the research lab because those pesky females had reproductive cycles or hormonal changes that could skew their results. And astonishingly, even for diseases more prevalent in women, most researchers have used male lab animals in their studies.[13]

One of the highlights (or lowlights) of the 2016 "Focused Cardiovascular Care for Women" report published in the journal *Mayo Clinic Proceedings (MCP)* was the revelation that very few if any hospitals offered focused cardiac care specifically for women before the year 2000. One reason for this may have been that, as the report's authors explained, "the concept of Women's Heart Clinics was met with hesitation from many cardiologists."[14]

Yes, you read that right. Until recently, it seems that the idea of establishing a women's heart clinic devoted to our unique physical complexities was not warmly welcomed by the physicians you'd think would be most supportive. Things are indeed changing, though. Women's heart clinics are now being established in major cities and teaching hospitals throughout North America and beyond.

The *MCP* report warns that, whether or not your community has a Women's heart clinic, recognizing that women are at significant risk of heart disease is not only important in providing appropriate care, but such recognition can avoid reflexively blaming women's symptoms on non-cardiac causes. The impressive report's female authors add:

The medical community in general, and women specifically, lack information on cardiovascular health and disease in women. This ignorance makes it less likely that women will receive guidance on

♥ preventing heart disease
♥ preventive strategies and referral for needed diagnostic testing
♥ appropriate treatment
♥ cardiac rehabilitation to help patients recover following treatment

Finally, the 2016 *MCP* report concludes with this blunt assessment: "The public health cost of misdiagnosed or undiagnosed cardiac disease in women is significant."

Are Diagnostic Errors in Cardiology Reported?

I'm often asked during my presentations on women's heart health what happens after patients with heart disease are misdiagnosed and thus not appropriately treated. Does that original misdiagnosis get reported? Do hospital administrators or department heads or senior attending physicians review the circumstances and figure out ways to avoid those diagnostic errors in caring for future patients? Is the misdiagnosis discussed as a case study teaching tool in medical school?

The answer is likely no, no, and no—other than perhaps a mention during informal staff conversations. As Emergency physician and broadcaster Dr. Brian Goldman once observed during his compelling TEDx talk ("Doctors Make Mistakes: Can We Talk about That?"), the three words that ER doctors most dread hearing from their colleagues are: "Do you remember?"[15]

Do you remember that patient you sent home . . . ?

I can't be 100 percent certain, of course, but I'm betting my next squirt of nitro spray that the Emergency physician who misdiagnosed me with acid reflux and sent me home despite those textbook heart attack symptoms did not voluntarily report this diagnostic error to his supervisor or to anybody else after I was correctly diagnosed during a later visit to the same hospital.

In 2015, the Institute of Medicine (IOM, now known as the National Academies of Sciences, Engineering, and Medicine) issued its long-awaited report called "Improving Diagnosis in Health Care." This report predicted that most adults will experience at least one diagnostic error in our lives, "sometimes with devastating consequences." But the document lacked any recommendation for health care professionals to report diagnostic errors, despite its clear call for "urgent change to address the potential danger to patients of such errors."[16]

Urgent change does not apparently include a recommendation for mandatory reporting of diagnostic errors, despite what the report calls "the pervasiveness of diagnostic errors and the risk for serious patient harm." Instead, this weak summary is offered up: "Voluntary reporting efforts should be encouraged and evaluated for their effectiveness."

I watched the IOM report launch briefing event live on my laptop screen, during which I heard this statement voiced twice by the report committee chair in response to media questions: "Now is not the right time for mandatory reporting of diagnostic errors."

The IOM report politely observes that, despite numerous calls for change, "efforts to improve voluntary reporting and analysis at the national level have been slow." So it looks like voluntary reporting of diagnostic errors isn't working. Why not, then, a clear recommendation for mandatory reporting of such errors, and why not now? If now is "not the right time" to require health care providers to report diagnostic errors, when might that right time be?

Meanwhile, out in the real world, mandatory reporting when bad things happen is entrenched in workplace culture in order to protect public safety. This movement explains why we no longer tolerate voluntary hard hat usage on construction sites, voluntary speed limit rules on our highways, or voluntary safety checklists by airline pilots before takeoff.

Let's imagine that the hospital that had sent me home with an acid reflux misdiagnosis had in place a policy that suggested its staff could (if they felt like it) voluntarily report such a diagnostic error as soon as that initial error became known to them (i.e., when I was later readmitted to the ER for correct diagnosis/treatment, or was found dead of a heart attack). I survived that heart attack despite being misdiagnosed during my first trip to the ER. I didn't die. I was still alive. So really, what's the harm? Did a diagnostic error ever happen if it was never reported?

Now let's imagine that a mandatory reporting protocol for diagnostic error had been in place that day (regardless of circumstance or outcome). As soon as the emergency medicine personnel during my second visit realized that I'd been previously misdiagnosed in the same ER on an earlier visit, an official reporting protocol could have helped staff record that this patient had been sent home earlier with a diagnostic error.

Dr. Pat Croskerry is a professor in emergency medicine at Dalhousie University in Nova Scotia, and widely considered among the world's foremost experts in diagnostic errors and patient safety. Here's how he explained two key areas of reporting improvement he's observed in his own hospital:

> When I first inherited the emergency department, we would have people presenting cases at rounds on their diagnostic triumphs. But we weren't looking critically at what we were doing. So we began focusing on cognitive errors, affective errors, biases, and distortions of reasoning. When I first came into my department, we were not doing that. It's been helped by the patient safety movement, of course, but there is now an openness and an honesty in the way that people will review their cases. That was one of our major gains.
>
> The other gain was that we really put a concerted effort into improving feedback. To have a system operating without feedback, as we often do in emergency departments, complex patients just disappear into the ICU or disappear into the morgue, and you haven't really learned anything. We implemented a number of strategies that have significantly improved our feedback.[17]

Providing that improved feedback loop after diagnostic error is all about trying to safeguard the health of future patients, just as protocols for workplace safety, highway safety, and aviation safety are seeking to protect future and potential victims of errors. Isn't it at last the right time to bravely declare that patients deserve the same measures to protect us, too? As the award-winning ProPublica journalist Marshall Allen warned his audience during his 2015 Medicine X presentation on patient safety at Stanford University: "Until you start measuring something, you can't improve it."[18]

4 ♡ The New Country Called Heart Disease

I am lying in a large and very white, bright, glass-walled room in the CCU (the coronary intensive care unit) of our local hospital. Two nurses are standing over me, one on either side of my bed, closely examining my right wrist. They're checking the wound that has been opened there in order to insert a catheter through the radial artery, up my arm, around the bend of my shoulder, and into my beating heart. I find it oddly touching that each of these women is gently holding one of my hands. I feel like weeping, and so I do.

I have no more pain. If anything, I'm simply feeling surprised. I have had a heart attack. I have had a heart attack! I, Carolyn Thomas, have had a frickety-frackin' heart attack. I now sport a stainless steel stent, a hollow tube resembling fine chicken wire, implanted into my left anterior descending coronary artery (LAD), one of the largest of the arteries feeding the heart muscle, the artery that was found to be 95 percent blocked.

I am also surprised that, although sedated, I've been able to watch the entire catheterization procedure live on a big screen overhead in the cath lab. That's my heart up there on the screen. My beating heart, squirts of contrast dye swooshing periodically into the catheter through my wrist, outlining my heart with every beat. But look—the interventional cardiologist performing the procedure points out to me one remarkable area of my heart where the dye is unable to get through. Blood flow in that part of the LAD artery simply seems to abruptly disappear. But then the angioplasty balloon is inserted, inflated, and oh!—another surprise, an involuntary scream of pain—while the balloon fully inflates and momentarily stops all blood flow to the heart muscle below that blockage. Within seconds, blessed relief as the balloon is deflated and swiftly removed from my body, leaving behind its perfectly placed stainless steel stent passenger. The stent will help to permanently prop open that once-blocked blood vessel, and will remain inside my heart for the rest of my life.

Another nurse walks into my glass box to ask if I'm hungry. A third surprise: she brings back a tray carrying a roast beef sandwich on white bread. This is what they serve people on a cardiac ward?

I make emotional phone calls to both of my children, each living out of town but now busy making plans to come home to be with their mother. I drift in and out of sleep. In between naps, I start eating my roast beef sandwich, and I decide I have never tasted anything more delicious.

Three visiting cardiology residents from Sweden interrupt my sandwich eating. They spend an hour or so interviewing me, asking many questions and taking careful notes. I ask them to remember my story when they go back home whenever they are tempted to dismiss Swedish women with classic heart attack symptoms because of what look like normal cardiac test results.

At one point during that first day in CCU, I am happy to see that two of my hospice colleagues are also waiting to see me. I spot the wide-eyed faces of Rod and Brenda near the nurses' station before they see me. They tiptoe carefully into my big glass box, and they seem uncharacteristically quiet.

I'm thinking that their faces reflect shock because I look better than they'd feared—or is it that I look really bad? I try to sit up a bit straighter in bed and paste on my best smiley face to reassure them. I don't know it yet, but I am soon going to be perfecting those pasted-on smiles, no matter how I'm feeling inside. Brenda explains that the news of my heart attack has rocketed through our workplace. They're anxious to catch up on every detail to report back to our hospice colleagues.

But the nurse returns to shoo them out of the CCU. Before they go, I ask them to tell Dave, our boss, that I might not be back at work tomorrow, but will most definitely be back on the day after that. I catch the eye-rolling as they leave.

Before I'm finally discharged from the hospital, I'm handed a prescription for a fistful of cardiac meds, which we'll pick up at the pharmacy on the way home.

And home is where the enormity of what has just happened to me begins to finally sink in.

What I Didn't Know before My Hospital Discharge

Not one person in the hospital's CCU asked me anything about who or what was waiting for me when I finally returned home. Was there anybody there, for example, who could help take care of me? Was there anybody at home I'd need to take care of? How much time off work would I be able to arrange in order to recuperate? Could I afford to pay for that fistful of expensive cardiac medications, most of which I would need to take for the rest of my natural life?

Not one person in the hospital advised me to prepare for the crushing fatigue that turns out to be very common in patients following a cardiac event. Not one practitioner warned me that post–heart attack depression is astonishingly common, yet treatable and temporary.

Not one person told me that heart disease is a chronic and progressive condition, and that even though my blocked coronary artery had been unblocked, doctors could not fix my heart disease.

Although all of the doctors and nurses I met in the hospital repeatedly asked about my possible cardiac risk factors (e.g., Do you have a family history of heart disease? Have you ever been a smoker?), not one of them asked if I'd ever experienced *pregnancy complications*. Such complications are known to be significant risk factors for later heart disease. I certainly didn't know back when I'd been diagnosed with preeclampsia while pregnant with Ben that the diagnosis meant I'd have two to three times the risk of having the heart attack that I eventually had. It was years later, in fact, that I learned about this personal risk factor, and only because I happened to read a *New York Times* interview with obstetrician and researcher Dr. Graeme Smith of Queen's University in Kingston, Ontario. Here's how he explained the link between pregnancy complications and heart disease:

"Pregnancy is the ultimate cardiac stress test. How much or how badly you fail that stress test really is an indicator of your future health risk. Pregnancy is a window of opportunity to screen women to ensure health preservation and heart disease prevention."[1]

The known association between heart disease and pregnancy complications (such as preeclampsia, gestational diabetes or gestational hypertension, miscarriage, full-term but low–birth weight baby, or pre-term birth) finally convinced the American Heart Association to start including pregnancy complications, for the first time ever, in the list of significant cardiac risk factors in its revised 2011 guidelines.[2]

Another bit of information I wasn't given before hospital discharge was how critically important it was to sign up for (and complete) a program of supervised *cardiac rehabilitation* in order to cut my mortality risk by two-thirds.[3] It turns out that the key predictor of cardiac rehab attendance is physician endorsement, although research suggests that an appallingly low number (as low as 20 percent) of eligible heart patients are actually referred by a physician to a supervised cardiac rehabilitation program.[4] Yet the known benefits of these programs are so important to heart patients that Mayo Clinic cardiologist Dr. Sharonne Hayes bluntly recommends: "If your doctor recommends cardiac rehabilitation, go. If you're not referred, ask. And if you ask and are told 'You don't need it,' find a new cardiologist."[5]

Doctors, please note: checking off a little tick box on a discharge form or clicking a button on a computer screen is not an endorsement. Physician endorsement means taking 12 seconds to say something like this out loud to your patient: "Cardiac rehabilitation is a terrific program for heart patients that has been proven to improve quality of life and significantly reduce your risk of dying from another cardiac event— and I strongly recommend that you complete this program."

Oregon cardiologist Dr. James Beckerman, author of the highly recommended book called *Heart to Start*, slams his colleagues who fail to refer their heart patients to cardiac rehab. "It is bad medicine to withhold life-saving treatments, and many physicians are selling their patients short. Cardiac rehabilitation is the best medication that you will never find in a television commercial, and its only side effect is a better quality of life."[6]

Not one person in the hospital told me to expect further chest pain once I was home, or how to deal with it if it happened. Not one person in the hospital sat me down with my new unopened canister of nitroglycerin and taught me the correct way to take this medication in case I suffered the chest pain of angina, as many new heart patients do. Each episode was terrifying. I learned how to do this on my own much later, when I discovered the writing of legendary cardiology pioneer Dr. Bernard Lown, who called this traditional medication "a wonder drug."[7] Nitro works to treat chest pain because it's a vasodilator, meaning it dilates coronary arteries and decreases the workload of the heart, both of which help to make heart patients with angina feel better.

Dr. Lown's best advice to heart patients on how to take nitroglycerin? At the first sign of angina, sit down, lean forward, inhale deeply, and bear down as if for a bowel movement before taking your nitro (either as a tablet or a spray). Wait five minutes, just sitting quietly. If pain persists, take another dose. Wait another five minutes. If pain still persists, you can take a third dose—but you'd better be calling 911 as you do.

Do not wait, as I did needlessly for months, until episodes of angina become increasingly severe before reaching for nitro relief. In fact, Dr. Lown urges heart patients living with angina to use it preventively. This practice was exemplified by a woman I met at Mayo Clinic who was a keen tennis player. She'd lived with chronic but stable angina for a long time, and it didn't slow her down. She would take a dose of nitro before beginning a game, and halfway through, she'd sit down for another dose, waiting a few minutes before picking up her tennis racket again. She'd done this day in and day out for years. Nitroglycerin, as I like to say, is your friend.

I learned that coming home didn't represent the end of my cardiac drama, but was instead merely the start of figuring out what else I needed to learn.

The Homecoming

Those first few days back at home were a blur, overwhelmingly busy with phone calls and a parade of visitors bearing food, cards, or flowers.

Six Personality Coping Patterns: Which One Are You?

In his excellent book *Heart Illness and Intimacy: How Caring Relationships Aid Recovery,* psychologist Dr. Wayne Sotile explores how our personalities and our coping patterns can often determine how we'll react to a life-changing cardiac event.[8]

Of these six basic personality coping patterns, which one are you?

1. *Being Strong:* People with this personality are taught to cope with life by being stoic and shouldering burdens without complaints or requests for help. Overwhelming or frightening situations (like having a heart attack) can fill them with shame and discomfort. Heart patients in this group are often in denial, and can suffer significant depression from the perception that others do not care, or they may focus on physical symptoms only as an indirect way to get support.
2. *Being Perfect:* Since perfection is never attained, those who are stuck in its pursuit may feel anxious, guilty, or never good enough, but may also believe that their internal anxiety will go away if only they can just do it perfectly. Heart patients in this group exhibit all or nothing self-critical thinking, like developing irritatingly rigid rules around their cardiac rehabilitation, and may worry obsessively about every detail of the illness.
3. *Trying Hard:* These personalities have learned to feel valued for their ability to try harder than the next person, for struggling longer and more tenaciously than others. They may have great difficulty determining when they have worked hard enough to deserve a rest, and may even feel anxious when they do try to relax or play. Heart patients in this group may feel demoralized and frustrated (with themselves and others) because of an excessive work ethic that interferes with enjoyment of everyday life.
4. *Pleasing Others:* These self-sacrificing folks think they've been put on Earth to take care of others, not themselves. It's

(continued)

hard for them to set appropriate limits for responding to the needs of others and expressing (or even identifying) their own important needs, so they often feel drained and martyred. They like to give to others the kind of attention and care they'd like to receive, but rarely ask directly for these gifts of love or attention. Heart patients in this group may go through recovery and rehabilitation feeling lonely, due to reluctance to express their emotional needs, and may also blame themselves excessively for the discomfort they cause in others by "putting the family through all this."

5. *Hurrying:* These personalities may feel uncomfortable, agitated, and frustrated with a reasonably paced lifestyle. They have become accustomed to an internal sense of urgency, and fill their lives with more to do than time allows, as if hurrying is necessary to survive. Heart patients in this group are similar to *Trying Hard* copers in their sense of urgency, but feel more frazzled or chaotic in response to the urgency, expressing frustration and irritability when they realize, for example, that cardiac rehabilitation is a lifelong process, not an event that will soon be finished. They may go for dangerous quick-fix cures, or just impatiently give up recommended heart health improvements.

6. *Being Careful:* Some people believe that living is a frightening proposition at best, filled with obsessive worrying and distressing anxiety in reaction to changes, big or small. They may doubt their own and others' abilities to cope with changes in the status quo, and have difficulty relaxing and enjoying themselves. Heart patients in this group sometimes suffer depression, questioning their own value as their self-esteem suffers during recovery and they become obsessive monitors, observers, and worriers who withdraw from life instead of trying to improve their quality of life.

Finally, no matter which coping pattern seems to fit either the heart patient or the patient's family members, Dr. Sotile suggests these four tips to help each other:

1. a basic understanding of each other's coping patterns
2. the courage to steer your own reactions in healthy directions
3. the perseverance to put up with discomfort until new coping patterns feel familiar
4. the loving support of family and friends while everybody learns new ways of reacting

Each new visitor meant telling and re-telling the details of the past several days. Lying back in my red reclining chair, surrounded by soft pillows and the plaid quilt my mother had given me years earlier, I often felt a bit like the royal family receiving official callers. I was moved by such an outpouring of caring support from family, friends, and neighbors, but I was also feeling utterly exhausted and overtaxed.

Some visitors were people I barely knew. One in particular was an acquaintance who phoned to tell me that she'd just heard the shocking news, felt absolutely terrible because of what I'd gone through, and insisted on coming over with a pan of lasagna. I had neither seen nor heard from this person in over 15 years—yet here she was, settling onto my living room couch while filling me in on more than a decade's worth of her family news. I was so tired that morning, I could barely keep my eyelids propped open, yet paradoxically was also too polite to summon the strength to ask her to stop talking and go home.

After that memorable visit, my family began to rethink the entire visitation business. They started fielding phone calls so I could nap. They took messages, gave out daily updates, and repeated firmly that, yes, Mom was allowed occasional visitors as long as the visits were brief. Very brief. My son Ben, for example, no longer offered to make tea or even take the coats of arriving guests. Instead, visitors stood hovering beside the red chair, staring at me for only as long as Ben deemed the minimally polite exposure, and were then duly thanked for their concern as he walked them back to the front door. Only a small number of our closest friends were invited to sit and stay—but even then, the family stopwatch was running.

My daughter Larissa, who lived out of town while attending college, had also flown home to help me. Her approach to caregiving was different from Ben's (which leaned toward reading aloud to me or picking out good movies for us to watch together). She instead sat down to review my entire patient take-home package, from wound care to medication side effects. She took copious notes and then went straight to work. She examined every inch of the fridge and kitchen cabinets, tossing out anything she deemed no longer suitable for a heart patient. She researched heart-healthy diets, made a grocery list, and then returned from shopping with armloads of food recommended in the well-studied Mediterranean diet.[9] She spent most days chopping, prepping, cooking, and packing up healthy meals for the freezer. Out of all of our family members, I think Larissa had been most frightened by this heart attack, and occasionally admonished, "Don't ever do this to me again!"

Both of my children discovered something else during their return home. They now had a serious cardiac risk factor that they'd never had before their mother's heart attack: a family history of heart disease. You, too, have such a risk factor if your mother or sister had a cardiac event before the age of 65, or if your father or brother had one before the age of 55. Grandparents, cousins, aunts, or uncles are not as important in determining this risk factor; only first-degree relatives (parents and siblings) count.

I recall that coming home from hospital was both wonderful and frightening. While still lying in the CCU, I'd been surrounded and monitored every moment by an entourage of experienced nurses and doctors who would know exactly what to do if anything went wrong. But as happy as I was to get home to the familiar surroundings I loved, I was now suddenly on my own, no matter how many family members or friends were right there with me. I'd been discharged from hospital with surprisingly little practical advice about what my life was about to look like next.

And Then the Homecoming Blues

When I was hospitalized for a full month as a teenager recuperating from a ruptured appendix and a nasty case of peritonitis, such long hospital stays were routine. But length of stay at hospitals has been steadily decreasing since the 1960s for many reasons, including advancements in medical technology, changes in clinical practice, and financial pressures on what hospital administrators call bed control. Most patients undergoing open heart surgery, for example, are typically sent home just three to five days post-op now. In determining hospital length of stay, the current emphasis seems to be on:

stabilizing the patient
minimizing the length of hospitalization
assigning further treatment and follow-up to an outpatient setting

Basically, shortening length of stay as much as humanly possible now appears to be the goal in most modern hospitals.

There can, of course, be certain advantages in speeding up hospital discharge times. Most of us would prefer to recuperate in a quiet space, sleep in our own beds, and consume decent food, far away from any possible contact with infectious hospital superbugs.

But for the freshly diagnosed heart patient, there can also be significant worries about leaving that reassuring 24/7 bubble of care. At home, experts are no longer checking in on us, bringing us meal trays, changing dressings, administering meds, or reassuring us when we have questions. Suddenly, we're back at home with people who have no medical training, and who may be even more worried about this scenario than we are.

It's not unusual for us to feel a fragile combination of anxiety and fear as we try to creep through this early adjustment period. Even the most routine task around the house may loom impossibly large. We long to get back to being the same independent people we were before all of this happened, yet we may not have even the slightest idea about what we can—or cannot—do anymore.

Women can feel especially shaken after returning home while we struggle to regain a sense of normalcy in the household. We sometimes feel shocked because we can't quite get our brains wrapped around this new reality, or resentful because after taking care of the whole family, we're the one who got sick.

Something else may strike during the first week or so, especially among family members of the heart patient. A type of coping overkill is linked, not surprisingly, to a new sense of fear that can cause families to turn into the heart health police, obsessed with catching the patient at the slightest failure to follow doctor's orders over even the most minor of daily decisions. Very few family members feel adequately prepared to provide appropriate care at home to a newly discharged heart patient.

Here's how Mayo Clinic experts describe this common patient reaction:

> After a traumatic event has occurred, you might need several days or weeks to fully process what has happened and come to grips with the challenges ahead. This type of denial can be a helpful response to stressful information. You initially deny the distressing problem. As your mind absorbs it, however, you can come to approach it more rationally over time.[10]

And when Virginia cardiac surgeon Dr. Marc Katz was a speaker at the annual Medicine X conference at Stanford University in 2013, he shared with his audience what often happens when we go from being just a person to being a heart patient:

> When people are given a serious cardiac diagnosis, many just shut down. They're scared to death, whether they admit it or not. They're afraid they might keel over with the next step, or that whatever horrendous procedure I'm going to recommend will disable them for the rest of their lives. I try to communicate to them: "Yes, this is a bad thing and I'm sorry you're in this circumstance, but here are the things we can do to help you."[11]

No matter what well-meaning reassurances physicians may offer, however, the reality for many of us is that time—and educating ourselves as much as possible—may ultimately be the best remedies to help us adjust to this new life. As I like to tell my women's heart health pre-sentation audiences, "Your only job now is to become the world expert in your own cardiac diagnosis."

Why Am I So Tired?

For my whole life BHA (Before Heart Attack), I can hardly remember feeling real fatigue. Oh, sure, I'd feel sore after working long sweaty days on our fruit farm as a teenager. Or sleepy after pulling all-nighters in college. Or out-of-my-mind exhausted trying to cope with a colicky infant and a teething toddler as a young mom. Or tired at the end of a stressful day juggling last-minute deadlines throughout my public re-lations career. Or maybe even pleasantly achy after my running group finished our long Sunday morning training runs.

But generally speaking, on a day-to-day basis, I'd never felt the kind of severe fatigue I experienced AHA (After Heart Attack). I wasn't expecting that fatigue like this was heading my way. I wasn't simply exhausted, I was becoming quite distressed by all of this exhaustion. What was wrong with me? Why wasn't I able to pull up my socks and just feel normal again?

I found surprising answers to those troubling questions in a Swed-ish study out of the University of Gothenburg. Researchers there found that about half of all patients who survive a heart attack are still expe-riencing "onerous fatigue" four months after diagnosis. Dr. Pia Alsén, lead author of this study, observed: "Many people recovering from heart attack experienced the fatigue as new and different, not related to phys-ical effort or a lack of rest; it occurred unpredictably and could not be attributed to any definite cause."[12]

It's hard to describe this kind of exhaustion to those who have never experienced it, or to explain fatigue that's not relieved by resting. This fatigue is not the same as feeling tired. It's more like having the flu, or being run over by a large bus.

The elusive reason for post–heart attack fatigue might also lie in the damage to the heart muscle caused by the heart attack itself, Dr. Alsén adds. When heart muscle is damaged by being deprived of oxygenated blood flow during a heart attack, scar tissue is formed, which can decrease the heart's efficiency, depending on the size and location of the damage. In my early days back at home, the simplest of tasks—even taking a shower—required a supreme effort and a 20-minute lie-down afterward to recover, during which I felt shaky, light-headed, and sick.

I remember going for a one-block walk with Ben shortly after coming home from the hospital. My post-op instructions from the CCU had been to walk outdoors one block a day for the first week, two blocks a day the second week, etc. By the way, I learned that such advice may have been too cautious, because it turns out that what a wounded heart might need most after a cardiac event is exercise. Some researchers now suggest that patients who begin a supervised exercise program one week after a heart attack have improved heart performance compared to patients who delayed exercising. In fact, for those who waited to begin exercise as I did, the results of delay seem dramatic, according to the University of Alberta's Dr. Mark Haykowsky; he found this surprising result in the heart patients he and his research team studied: "For every week that new heart patients delayed starting their exercise treatment, they would have to train for the equivalent of one month longer to get similar benefits."[13]

Back to that eventful one-block walk: Ben and I had barely made it as far as the stop sign at the end of our block when I had to grab his arm to lean on for support all the way home. I couldn't believe it! I felt like a frail old lady, scarcely able to shuffle one foot in front of the other. And when we finally returned home (slowest walking pace in recorded history), I collapsed in a heap to recuperate, already wondering if I should just avoid walking entirely.

But it turns out that, despite my tiredness, Ben was right to encourage me to get outside for those walks every day, each day going a bit farther. And unless specifically instructed by your physician to rest, as Dr. Haykowsky's team reported, what generally helps the wounded heart is work, not rest.

So what can we do when fatigue makes it hard to follow such advice? Over the years, my always-generous *Heart Sisters* blog readers have shared these tips that might also work for you, especially during those fragile early days:

♥ Take it nice and slow.

♥ Get out of bed at the same time each morning.

♥ Guard your energy, especially in the first few weeks.

♥ You have nothing to prove, and there is no prize for doing too much, too fast.

♥ Try to maintain a regular schedule for bedtime with a quiet, no-screen routine beforehand.

♥ Perfect the art of taking 20-minute naps.

♥ Get outside every single day to breathe fresh air.

♥ Pay attention to eating healthy foods on a regular schedule.

♥ Watch your consumption of caffeine and sugar.

♥ Try relaxation, gentle stretching, or meditation techniques.

♥ Plan your day carefully. Alternate periods of activity and rest.

♥ While resting, plan for what you'll do when you are more able.

♥ Check for side effects of medicines. Take them at the best time of day to minimize side effects (for example, if fatigue or dizziness are known side effects, ask if you can take those before bedtime).

♥ Accept the reality that your usual To Do list will not be accomplished today.

♥ Respect your recovering body, what it can do today, and what it can't.

♥ Watch a funny movie. It won't make you less tired, but laughing will make you feel better.

Exercise physiologists often refer to fatigue caused by daily activities by using measurements they call METs (or *metabolic equivalents of task*).[14] Different activities are assigned different MET ratings depending on how much physical energy they require. One MET is basically the energy it takes just to sit quietly. The higher the METs, the more energy the activity takes. METs numbers can range from 1 (sitting, for example) to 10.0 (jumping rope).

Here are some other common daily activities and their MET scores:

Driving a car	2.0
Walking 3 mph	3.0
Showering	3.5
Sex	3.7–5.0
Golfing	4.0
Gardening	4.5
Playing tennis	6.0
Cross-country skiing	8.0[15]

In the very early days of recuperating following a cardiac event, our doctors may ask us to take it easy by avoiding activities that require more than about 3 METs. Taking a shower, for example, scores a 3.5 on the METs scale. No wonder showering felt so tiring at first! Showering can include raising the arms to shampoo our hair. Raising both arms above the head can sometimes place an extra workload on the heart known as the pressor response—particularly for those not used to working out.[16]

Accepting—and Offering—Help

When I was newly home from the hospital after my heart attack, I appreciated kindhearted friends and family who said, "Just call me if there's anything at all that I can do for you!"

But, frankly, I knew that I was not going to call them to ask:

"Can you come over and change the kitty litter?"

That was never going to happen.

I often felt reluctant to ask directly for help, even when I most needed it. Didn't want to be a bother, didn't want to make a fuss, didn't want to sound like an invalid. I also undoubtedly wanted to be back to my old self—the self who could lift heavy objects, multi-task, and clean out the damned kitty litter box. So when people gave specific offers (such as calling to say, "I'm at the grocery store—what can I pick up for you while I'm here?," for example), it didn't feel so much like a direct request.

If you are, as I was, reluctant to put others to any trouble, remember how satisfying it has felt for you when you've been able to pitch in to help somebody in need. Don't deprive those who care about you from helping you out when you most need it, too, and when they most need to feel helpful.

If you're looking for ways to be helpful to people who are newly diagnosed with almost any serious condition, or are sick in bed or incapacitated compared to how they are in their usual lives, I've come up with some suggestions.

But first, here's my list of tips on what to avoid doing or saying:

♥ Don't start in on that story of your Uncle Stan and his much more interesting heart attack; the freshly diagnosed simply do not care about other people's medical drama at this moment.

♥ Don't try to push any life-saving miracle cures, products, or supplements on us, particularly if you are selling them (this is unforgivably tacky).

♥ Don't try to cheer us up if we're having a bad day. We're entitled to have a bad day once in a while because we've just had a frickety-frackin' heart attack—and if we do one day confess that we are feeling low or scared or sick, do not say things like, "Well, at least you look good!" unless you want to hear us muttering, "If you only knew . . ." You don't need to fix anything.

♥ Don't suddenly stop helping. People are generally quick to come forward to offer help in the early days soon after hearing about another person's health crisis, but it's common to lose interest over time. Keep offering the help you gave at the time of your friend's initial diagnosis until the person tells you to stop. If you're unable to continue, at the very least, stay in touch.

♥ Here are some phrases to avoid entirely:
Stay positive!
Dr. Oz / Jenny McCarthy / Gwyneth Paltrow recommends _____.
All you need to do is _____.
You're taking too much medicine.
It's all in your head.
Aren't you feeling better yet?

Now here are some other suggestions of things to do that might actually be helpful:

♥ Always check first before you assume the patient is comfortable with you pitching in to help (watching you sort her dirty underwear for the laundry may not make her feel comfortable). If she declines your offer, don't take it personally. This is not about you.

♥ A sick person, like healthy people, may sometimes just want to be alone. If you repeatedly offer help or visits but are repeatedly turned down, take the hint and don't persist in volunteering. Send a nice card or flowers to let her know you're wishing her well.

♥ Keep your visits brief at first. I can't stress this enough. Just making conversation, even with people we love, can feel exhausting for us, especially at the beginning of our healing when we need to rest. Check with your friend's preferences, but generally, short visits are easiest to manage.

♥ Patients, don't be shy about asking for what you really want when it comes to visitors. If what you really want is no visitors outside of family, tell the truth. Tell others you'd prefer they wait to visit until you are starting to feel better. One of my blog readers told me this story: "The hospital chaplain came to my room during my last hospital stay and asked me if I had anyone in my life. My answer was I have too many, and at times like these, I cannot handle their drama. I am simply not strong enough and need to put all my energy into my own healing."

♥ Visitor guidelines also apply to hospital visitors. Most hospitals now have wide-open (read: non-existent) visiting hours. Personally, I'm not a fan of these relaxed visiting restrictions for non-family members, especially during the early days when we're tired and just need to doze off frequently. Some patients love having company, and some prefer nobody around them except for immediate family, so don't assume your visit will be welcomed at this time. And some facilities don't allow children or pets to visit, so always ask first.

♥ After hospital discharge, remember that gifts of service or time are almost always a good idea. For example, one friend came over and planted all my summer annuals for me because she knew I was not able to do that; another called to say he was coming over to wash, vacuum, and gas up the little green car. Some people may need someone to pick up their mail, help the spouse with the kids, or provide rides to school or medical appointments. Try to anticipate what needs doing that might be hard for a sick person to do.

♥ Food! Offer to bring a heart-smart casserole, soup, vegetarian chili, or (best idea ever!) a big fresh salad when you visit. Offer some choices like: "I'm bringing your lunch over on Saturday: sandwiches or sushi?"

♥ If you're part of a group of people who are all close to the person, consider pooling your resources. One of my blog readers told me that her co-workers chipped in to have three dinners a week delivered from a local caterer during her recuperation. Another wrote that her book club members funded a weekly housecleaning service for her first month post-op. And another was thrilled when the women in her walking group walked over every week with a fresh fruit tray for her (very handy idea because when you do have visitors, you'll always have something healthy to snack on).

♥ Pick out a special magazine you think the person would enjoy.

♥ Bring a stack of library books selected just for her (one of my neighbors, for example, brought over six gorgeous library books on flower-arranging—which she knew was a keen interest of mine—and then made a plan to return them all to the library for me before the due date).

♥ Offer to drive the person to appointments—or just out for tea. Many heart patients are restricted from driving for a specified time after hospital discharge.

♥ Consider the kind of relationship you already have with the person who's been diagnosed. Remember that story of the woman I hadn't seen in 15 years who camped out on my couch for painful hours right after I came home from the hospital? Don't be that woman. Many patients have reported that they're sometimes surprised either by the close friends who seemed to abandon them during a medical crisis, or by casual acquaintances who stepped in as if you two now enjoyed a level of intimacy you've never shared. Both options can cause discomfort. Few things in life are more disappointing than when someone we care about isn't there for us when we really need them, and conversely, we can feel awkward being on the receiving end of a one-sided brand-new relationship. Always check with the person first.

♥ Ask the person to make a Job Jar for you, filled with notes about suggested errands, big or small, that need doing. When we're feeling really sick, we may feel unable to tackle even the smallest task, yet these are often what we worry about the most if they're not getting done. Is that rosebush getting enough water today? Am I running out of toilet paper? Do I need to mail my sister's birthday card by Tuesday? These could all be Job Jar tasks. Visitors can reach into the jar to pull out one or two pieces of paper listing very specific small tasks they can help with.

♥ If the person lives alone, or with a spouse who's away at work all day, you could offer to do regular tasks on a regular schedule if you can (walking the dog, mowing the lawn, picking up the kids, watering houseplants, helping with laundry, or pitching in with those Job Jar errands). This suggestion also has the benefit of giving an overwhelmed spouse a break, too.

♥ If you're especially close to a sick person, you can offer to set up a free page at CaringBridge.org or CareCalendar.org for her. These non-profit websites will allow her or a loved one to share health updates (so she won't have to keep fielding daily calls from all those people checking up on her), and it also lets friends/family sign up to schedule help with chores and errands.

♥ Remember anniversaries. Patients seldom forget the day they were diagnosed, the day they were admitted to the hospital, or the day they began/finished treatment. Every May 6, I have a touching little *Heart-iversary* moment to mark a significant outcome (I'm still here!). Make a note to remember your friend's milestone date, too.

Above all, even if you do none of the above, remember that perhaps the kindest and most helpful thing you can do for somebody struggling with a new diagnosis is to simply be a willing and patient listener.

Welcome to Your New Country

My family doctor once compared my uneasy adjustment since suffering a heart attack to being like a stressful move to a foreign country.

I used to be pretty comfortable in my old country, pre–heart attack. I was healthy, active, outgoing. I had a wonderful family and close friends, a meaningful public relations career I loved, a condo renovated top to bottom in a charming leafy neighborhood of the most beautiful city in Canada—and a busy, happy, regular life.

Then on May 6, 2008, the day I was finally hospitalized for that widow maker heart attack, I moved far, far away to a different country. I couldn't speak the language, I didn't know the culture, and I had no map to find my way back home.

Exiled to this foreign country called Heart Disease, I found that nothing around me felt familiar or normal anymore. I was in a profound state of denial and shock. I was afraid of every odd twinge my body experienced. I also felt deeply ashamed—and shocked—because I just could not seem to pull myself together. I couldn't understand why I was still having ongoing cardiac symptoms, and neither could my doctors. I was quickly using up all my vacation days and banked sick time hours at work, but with no relief in sight and ongoing symptoms that were keeping me from going back to work.

What was wrong with me? Why wasn't I able to just snap out of it?

One day, weeks after the heart attack, I felt like I had had quite enough of being a patient, thank you very much. In a fit of pique, I marched around the apartment gathering up get-well cards and bouquets of flowers and anything else reminding me that some kind of invalid lived here. I tossed all of them into the trash, and waited to feel better.

It didn't work.

I was seeing my physician on a weekly basis by now, had to go back into the hospital for another cardiac procedure, was newly diagnosed with inoperable *coronary microvascular disease* (MVD), was referred to the regional pain clinic to address what doctors call *refractory angina* (chest pain that doesn't respond to usual medical treatments), and was prescribed drugs to help get me through this overwhelming state of pain and worry.

But as Susannah Fox, Chief Technology Officer at the US Department of Health and Human Services, once wrote for the Pew Internet Center:

> It's not surprising that when someone gets dropped into this kingdom of the sick, they grab their phones, they grab their laptops, they grab their loved ones, and they go. They go into that unfamiliar area of a new diagnosis, a new drug, a new treatment. They consult experts. They call and search and text. They band together and form posses, pioneers sharing maps with newcomers.[17]

That's what I did, too.

To try to make sense out of something that made no sense to me, I began to research women's heart disease like I was cramming for a cardiology midterm. I tried to figure out why an experienced ER physician had sent me home with an acid reflux misdiagnosis despite my textbook heart attack symptoms, and why so many other women were being misdiagnosed, too.[18] While looking up answers to these questions on the Mayo Clinic website one morning, I learned about the WomenHeart Science and Leadership Symposium for Women with Heart Disease held each year at Mayo in Rochester.

Hey! I'm a woman with heart disease! I decided to apply for this prestigious training program, intrigued by two key factors. The first, of course, was the opportunity to be awarded an all-expenses-paid trip to the world-famous Mayo Clinic to learn everything I possibly could about women's heart health. The second was based on my geographical ignorance, namely my belief that Rochester's proximity to my mother's home near Niagara Falls, New York, would allow me to stop over to visit Mom while I was basically in the neighborhood.

A few months later, I became the first Canadian ever accepted to attend this top-notch community educator training. That's also when

I learned that Mayo is not actually situated in Rochester, New York, but among the vast cornfields surrounding Rochester, Minnesota— nowhere near my mother's neighborhood.

Going to Mayo Clinic in October of 2008 was a life-changing experience. For starters, I was surrounded by 45 other women, all living with heart disease. The faculty of female cardiologists who steered our intensive curriculum turned out to be the rock stars of cardiology. After returning home to the West Coast, I began speaking to women about what I'd just learned at Mayo. As my health allowed, I started with small groups of 20 to 25 women at what I called my Pinot & Prevention events.

The Mayo Clinic reputation also opened doors for me through invitations to speak about what I'd learned there to health care professionals in mental health, cardiology, emergency medicine, and other medical specialties. Six months later, I launched my blog, *Heart Sisters*.[19] My public relations friends tease me that this is just what happens when a PR person has a heart attack. We keep on doing what we've always done, the only things we know how to do: writing and speaking and looking stuff up.

In this new country called Heart Disease, the culture demands a profound respect for pacing (a skill I had not ever bothered to master). This means learning new customs, like putting myself and my physical/mental/emotional health needs first. This seems to be harder than you'd think, particularly for women. It means learning how to nap like a preschooler, or just to sit and have a rest when I need to. It means learning to limit social contact to those who lift my spirits, make me laugh, or bring me casseroles. It means learning how to say "No!" to a lot of things, from Tim Hortons Maple Dip doughnuts to those "energy vampire" people who can suck the life right out of you.

At first it was extremely painful, as a recently arrived citizen in this new country, to learn that those still living in my old country of the well were doing just fine without me. As the old saying goes, "The graveyards of the world are filled with indispensable people." Or again, from Susannah Fox: "The number one thing that people try to do is to get the hell out of the kingdom of the sick and back to the kingdom of the well."[20]

The reality, however, is that some of us have been forced to permanently surrender our passports and will not ever get back.

Welcome to your new country.

5 ♡ Depressing News about Depression and Heart Disease

As the first few post–heart attack weeks pass, I begin to feel a cold creeping daily angst around how I should be feeling by now.

I have just survived what many do not. Shouldn't I be feeling happy and grateful because I am alive, because I'm lucky enough to live a few blocks from world-class cardiac care, because I have a strong social support network of family and friends around every day to fuss over me?

I often feel a mix of both crushing fatigue and anxiety at the same time, convinced by unusual bouts of ongoing chest pain and shortness of breath that a second heart attack must be imminent. It feels like low-grade terror on a daily basis. Every sudden new twinge makes me pause and wonder, "Is this something? Is it nothing? Should I call 911?"

My worried family and friends can't even begin to comprehend what's going on for me—I can scarcely understand it myself. I learn to smile my best PR smiles around them so we can all pretend that everything is getting better. "I'm fine, just fine."

But I'm overwhelmed, frightened, and confused—and certainly too ashamed to tell anybody the truth about how I'm really feeling. I've already put my family through so much because of my cardiac event. How can I add to that burden by not being and sounding better? Surrounded by all of their affectionate concern, how dare I feel anything but a good patient's appropriately cheerful dose of gratitude?

I begin to frighten myself by weeping openly over nothing in particular. I have no interest in reading, walking, talking. I can't seem to concentrate on anything. I sleep in my clothes, and when dawn comes, it's almost impossible to drag my dead-tired self out of bed.

Making even minimal conversation feels so tiring that it ultimately seems much easier to just avoid other people entirely. I start making excuses when friends, neighbors, or co-workers call to ask about going out or dropping by for a visit. "Maybe later in the week?"

I no longer seem to care how I look or how I smell. I'm puzzled by this new attitude, but not puzzled enough, based on results, to start caring. One morning, for example, before a follow-up appointment with my family doctor, I am having a very hard time trying to decide whether or not I should wash my hair.

Normally, showering and hair-washing are just part of my regular daily routine—not something to be decided upon at all. But on this particular day, some part of me knows that this might be the third or fourth or maybe even the fifth day in a row I've gone without bothering to shower, and maybe I shouldn't let my doctor know this. I wouldn't want her to see how bad things have become for me. Wouldn't want her to see me without my perfectly normal smile/makeup/clothes/hair.

When I break down crying in her office later that morning (hair finally washed and even a brave smear of lipstick on), she seems genuinely surprised by this uncharacteristic outburst. She tries to buck me up by reminding me that she's known me for over 30 years, she knows what a strong person I've always been, and furthermore, she feels extremely confident that I will detour right past this little bump in the road with no trouble at all. "Can't you just push through it?" she asks.

I can see that even this person, this person who has been our family doctor for decades, seems to neither understand nor approve. I fish in the bottom of my purse for tissues, pull myself together, return to that smiley face, and somehow manage to walk out of her office.

But back at home, I collapse. I am filled with despair. I also feel deeply ashamed that, despite my doctor's little cheerleading lecture, I don't seem able to pull myself together. And no, I can't just push through this.

Before falling exhausted into bed later, I start cleaning. I wipe counters and sweep floors, straighten bath towels and empty recycling bins. I must tidy up in case I die in my sleep and the paramedics (or worse, my family) have to come in tomorrow morning and discover my body. It somehow seems important that they find the corpse in a nice tidy apartment. I'm doing this every night. Night after night, I am consciously preparing for my own death.

The upside of this kind of anxiety: the apartment has never looked so good.

But worst of all, none of this feels like my real self anymore, like my real life, my real world. I begin to worry that the old Carolyn has truly disappeared. What if I'm unable to ever get her back?

How Situational Depression Hurts Heart Patients

I don't think I ever actually used the word depression to describe to my doctor or to anybody else how I was feeling in those awful early weeks. I knew nothing about depression. I just knew that something was terribly wrong with me. Why couldn't I just will myself to snap out of whatever this was?

The type of depression that persists after a serious health crisis like a heart attack is often known as situational depression or stress response syndrome. It's what mental health professionals describe as an adjustment disorder that can strike within weeks following a traumatic life event as we struggle to make sense of something that makes no sense.

Dr. Stephen Parker is a cardiac psychologist in Alaska who also happens to be a multiple heart attack survivor himself. He's blunt in his professional assessment of the known link between a cardiac event and subsequent depression.

> There are damned good reasons to feel anxious and depressed. Who the hell wouldn't get depressed and anxious after a heart attack? A heart attack is a deeply wounding event, and it is a wound that can take a long time to recover from, whatever the treatment.
>
> Depression after a heart attack essentially forces the person to rest, to take time to re-evaluate one's life and the road that led to the heart attack, to use all available energy and resources for healing, both physically and psychologically.
>
> I personally recommend being very depressed after a heart attack, sleeping a lot, taking it easy, not expecting much of yourself. Be lost for a while.[1]

He has also observed that a serious cardiac diagnosis is almost always accompanied by what he calls the "swirling emotions of heart disease." These include:

relief at survival
disbelief and anger that this has happened
grief for everything that has and will be lost
gratitude to those who helped
extreme vulnerability in a previously safe world
fear of what the future might bring

Psychologist Dr. Elvira Aletta, director of Explore What's Next and author of *Seven Rules for Living Well with Chronic Illness,* often uses the word grief to describe the symptoms experienced by patients newly diagnosed with a chronic illness like heart disease. She explains that this new grief is often piled on top of the regular kinds of daily grief, big or small, that we all live with.

> Chronic illness means getting sick and being told it is not going away, and that stinks. Our bodies have suddenly freaked out on us, and we've lost control of the one thing we thought we could count on.
>
> There are so many ways life almost kills us. The responsibility of caring for elderly parents, a disabled child, a spouse. The burden of being a single parent. Discovering that the person you thought you could trust with your most precious heart turns out to be unworthy. Losing a loved one to illness or death, slowly or suddenly. Being worn down looking for a job or being in a job you hate. Fighting for our own lives when sickness strikes and doesn't politely go away like it's supposed to. All of the above happening all at once.
>
> Trauma, emotional dark pits, cascading series of unfortunate events. They happen. Life happens.

And some days, as Dr. Aletta reminds us, we just have to rage. "Cry, whine, moan, pout, eat ice cream right out of the carton or whipped cream straight from the aerosol can!"[2]

In between all that crying and whining and moaning and pouting (and yes, eating ice cream right out of the carton just as Dr. Aletta recommends), I started practicing how to look and sound like the old me.

I tried to laugh like the old Carolyn used to laugh, I tried to talk like the old Carolyn did, I tried to listen and nod and smile around other people in the same familiar way that the old Carolyn would have done.

But ongoing, untreated depression remains a potentially dangerous condition if you're a heart patient, because we know that people struggling with depression are far less motivated to:

- ♥ take their daily cardiac medications as prescribed
- ♥ exercise regularly
- ♥ adopt a heart-healthy diet
- ♥ quit smoking
- ♥ avoid social isolation
- ♥ show up for medical appointments or cardiac rehabilitation classes
- ♥ follow basic medical recommendations that will aid recuperation and reduce the risk of having another cardiac event[3]

Dr. Colleen Norris is a cardiac researcher studying female patients who have developed symptoms of depression following a heart attack. Her research, published in the *European Journal of Cardiovascular Nursing,* found that 74 percent of women living with depression following a cardiac event still had impaired physical and social functioning one year after that heart attack. That impairment also meant that women's overall recovery, independence, and quality of life were significantly impacted. Dr. Norris also noted that women can feel under pressure to return immediately to work and to their usual relentless role of family caregiver, instead of accepting the fact that they are the ones who may need care during the early weeks and months of recovery. She added, "It is so important that we start addressing the depressive status if we wish to see improvements in outcomes of our female patients with coronary artery disease."[4]

The age of a heart patient may also be an important factor here. Dr. Susmita Mallik of Emory University School of Medicine reported in the *Archives of Internal Medicine* that women diagnosed with heart disease before the age of 60 are three times more likely to become depressed than their male counterparts are. Dr. Mallik warned, "Both doctors and patients should be aware that depression is an important risk factor for adverse outcomes for cardiac event survivors."[5]

Depression, the Often-Overlooked Cardiac Problem

Some heart patients may already have a history of depression that started long before they were diagnosed with a cardiac condition (and pre-existing depression is in fact a known heart disease risk factor).[6] There's a disturbing link between women's heart disease and depression. Those suffering depression are more at risk for developing heart disease, and those diagnosed with heart disease are more at risk for suffering depression. Many, like me, can become newly depressed for the first time ever as an acute reaction to a traumatic diagnosis.

If you're a recovering heart patient, you may wish that somebody had warned you that this kind of situational depression after a cardiac event is not only predictable, but is almost always temporary and treatable. Wouldn't it make sense for physicians to monitor and address these common symptoms early on, instead of labeling us as non-compliant when we stop following doctor's orders because we feel so bad?

But some heart specialists may have neither enough time nor expertise to address depression in their freshly diagnosed patients, according to Mayo Clinic's Dr. Sharonne Hayes: "Cardiologists may not be comfortable with touchy-feely stuff," she explained. "They want to treat lipids and chest pain. And most are not trained to cope with mental health issues."[7]

Despite what we know about how dangerous depression can be following a cardiac event, it turns out that researchers have been reporting on unrecognized depression in heart patients for more than 40 years, according to Dr. David L. Hare. In his 2014 historical review of depression and cardiovascular disease, he reported that symptoms of depression are found in up to 60 percent of patients after an acute heart attack, with major clinical depression identified in about 15 percent of them. These numbers are two to three times higher than the depression statistics found among the general population.[8]

However, the subject of depression associated with heart disease isn't being overlooked everywhere. Consider, for example, that the official cardiology treatment guidelines published by the European Society of Cardiology recommend to all member cardiologists that heart patients should be "routinely screened for signs of depression."[9]

Yet generally speaking, depression in heart patients has "flown under the radar for far too long," concludes Dr. Colleen Norris. Like the European cardiac guideline authors, she and her research team now urge doctors to be alert for symptoms of depression in patients undergoing treatment for any form of heart disease, and particularly in their female patients.[10]

Not all feelings of sadness qualify as depression. Many of us have temporary feelings of sadness after experiencing different life events while we try to process what's just happened to us, and what we fear we've lost. This sadness typically diminishes very gradually within a few weeks for most heart patients as we are slowly able to adapt, and as we resume normal routine and activities.

Sometimes, however, it isn't just sadness, and a depressed mood following a cardiac event can be accompanied by other debilitating signs over a prolonged period of time:

- ♥ withdrawal from regular activities
- ♥ not responding when around family and friends
- ♥ increased negative thoughts and tearfulness
- ♥ no interest or pleasure in things we used to enjoy
- ♥ crying for no reason at all
- ♥ trouble thinking, remembering, or focusing on what we're doing
- ♥ just not caring
- ♥ sleeping all the time, yet feeling exhausted

This list is pretty well the exact description of my own symptoms. If these signs persist every day for two to three weeks, or get worse over time, you need to seek help. Please do not make the decision to wait in misery, as I did, for your physician or somebody else to intervene.

Sometimes, even those who are trained in mental health issues might not be as straightforward as they could be in giving us a "heads up" about this common problem. For example, two months after hospital discharge, at the final class of our seven-week "Heart to Heart" patient education classes for freshly diagnosed heart patients, the guest speaker was the cardiac social worker at our local hospital. She talked openly about psychological issues associated with heart disease. Feelings of depression and anxiety, she explained, are frequently experienced after a cardiac diagnosis. She listed the depression symptoms listed above, word for word, that are often reported by heart patients.[11]

I'd experienced all of them. I recall feeling a bizarre glimmer of what felt like hope as she spoke that evening, because I finally realized that I wasn't the only one feeling this way. Over two months of suffering, and everything she was confirming about situational depression in heart patients was news to me.

Why, I asked our guest speaker after class that evening, isn't this important topic right up front at the beginning of our seven-week schedule of topics? Why make us wait seven long weeks, during which time I'd pretty well convinced myself I was going crazy?

"Might scare people off," she replied.

I Finally Ask for Help

After hearing the social worker's very helpful talk at that Heart to Heart class, I decided I needed to speak to my family physician again. I told her what we'd learned during that class, that depression symptoms are frequently reported among heart patients, and that treatments such as talk therapy, medications, and others can make a big difference. I asked her for a referral to a mental health professional to help me work through all this.

"There's a one-year waiting list for a psychotherapy consultation," my doctor responded flatly. One year? I felt crushed. I honestly didn't know if I could even survive a whole year feeling this awful. I began weeping and was embarrassed to find that I couldn't seem to stop this time.

My physician handed me a piece of paper and asked me to complete a survey. It was a tick box list of the depression symptoms that the

Non-drug Ways to Treat Depression in Heart Patients

What else could those living with depressive symptoms be doing—with or without pharmaceutical help? Here are six non-drug options:

1. Talk Therapy: I found my own visits to a therapist tough at first, but profoundly helpful in adjusting to the new normal of living with heart disease. The two most commonly used talk therapies for depression are cognitive-behavioral therapy and interpersonal therapy. The former focuses on identifying how our negative thought patterns can affect how we feel; the latter focuses on how we relate to others. Both types of therapy can be effective.

2. Exercise: This has been found to be among the most effective treatments for depression. A brisk 30-minute walk, bike ride, or swim can also raise the body's level of serotonin, a brain chemical that affects mood and social behavior.

3. Watch Your Comfort Habits: Mindless consumption of coffee, alcohol, sugar, and recreational drugs may feel good temporarily, but these can aggravate mood disorders.

4. Sunlight: For some people, the shortening days of late autumn and winter are the beginning of a type of depression called seasonal affective disorder (SAD), which can last until spring. Try spending more time outdoors during the day, and arrange your environment so that you receive maximum sunlight. Many people with SAD respond well to exposure to light therapy that involves sitting beside a specially designed light box for several minutes a day. Consult your physician before beginning light therapy.

5. Regular Human Contact: Sometimes, people feel depressed because they are isolated, and they're isolated because they feel so depressed. This is a tough dilemma when the only thing we really feel like doing is hiding under the covers, all day, every day. But counting on our friends, neighbors, and family for regular companionship—even if just a short outdoor

(continued)

walk—can actually help to lift our spirits and get us through one day at a time.

6. Challenge Your Thinking: When things go wrong, we might have a tendency to exaggerate the consequences and imagine that results will always be disastrous. This may not be true at all. This is sometimes known as catastrophizing. Try asking, "What would I tell a friend if she or he had the same thoughts?" or "Am I confusing possibility with certainty?" or "Have I confused a thought with an actual fact?"

cardiac social worker had told us about. Check. Check. Check. And check. My doctor wrote me a prescription for antidepressant medication and told me that it may take a while for these meds to take effect, but that most people start to feel some benefit in three to six weeks.

I returned to see her later for a follow-up visit as required, but wasn't able to report that I was feeling much improvement, if any. She pulled out her prescription pad again, and told me that she wanted to start me on a different drug that might work better for me. Weeks and then months went by, with many medication prescription tweaks. Each follow-up appointment meant another stab at the depression survey.

By now, I had discovered an online support group run by Women-Heart: The National Coalition for Women with Heart Disease, part of the huge *Inspire* website patient community. I'd already found some comfort learning from dozens of discussion topics and thousands of women on that cardiac site who seemed to understand what I was going through.[12] I knew I couldn't tell my family or friends the same things that I could share with these heart patients, or ask the many questions I had. As much as my family and friends cared about me, what they really wanted and needed was for me to be okay again. "I'm fine, just fine." Nobody on the WomenHeart site expected me to be anything other than who I was.

I knew instinctively that I could benefit from a face-to-face support group if only there were one available in our community (there wasn't at that time, but I'm happy to say that there is now an active Women-Heart monthly support group held at our local hospital). You can find out if there's one near you by checking the WomenHeart website.[13]

I knew that the role of a professional therapist was to both listen and to offer tools to help us gain perspective. That's what I needed, no matter how long the waiting list.

Most importantly, I also knew I needed my family physician's referral to get an appointment with a therapist. So at my next doctor's appointment, I asked politely if she remembered my first referral request long ago, adding that if she had agreed to refer me back then, I'd have already moved up that long waiting list by now.

I could tell that, for whatever personal or professional reason, she was not keen on providing a psychotherapy referral. Period. Instead, she suggested we give the antidepressant drugs more time to work, or switch antidepressants again, or increase the drug dosage. It seemed clear to me that she was willing to offer anything—except that professional referral for non-drug talk therapy.

But this time, I persisted. She finally sighed, pulled out a contact list of mental health resources from the back of her desk drawer, and said to me, "Well, I suppose that you want to see a good one." I'm guessing now that, had I not felt so dreadful, I may have laughed out loud at that preposterous statement. No, I'd prefer to see a bad one, thanks . . .

My physician (also known as my former physician) told me she'd have to fax referral requests to a number of the mental health professionals on her list, because this very long waiting list meant that a multiple shotgun approach was the only way to find even one therapist in this entire city who would be able to squeeze me in at some point in the distant future.

A few days later, I returned home from a trip to the grocery store to find five phone messages waiting. Each was from a different psychotherapist's office in town, offering me an immediate consultation appointment that same week. I arbitrarily picked a counselor whose office was within walking distance from home, and one day later I was sitting on her couch.

One. Day. Later.

I had been suffering for months, not even guessing that my doctor had been quite wrong in her dismissive "one-year waiting list" claim.

My experience is a cautionary tale in a number of ways. First, it's an illustration of how tough it can be for a new heart patient to assertively ask for help while feeling fragile, sick, and overwhelmed. Second, it illustrates how valuable the art of persistence can be, and how we shouldn't give up on those gut feelings about what we really need. And third, it also illustrates that we can't always believe what we hear.

When I was at Mayo Clinic, I was shocked to learn there that fewer than 10 percent of heart patients are appropriately identified by their health care providers as needing psychological support for depression.[14]

While the situational depression associated with heart disease may respond well to pharmaceutical help, there are a number of non-drug options to consider—like that psychotherapist's appointment I was finally able to book. There's a clear mind-body connection here. While depression can show up as physical symptoms such as sore muscles, headache, or aching joints, regular physical exercise has also been shown to be surprisingly effective in those diagnosed with depression. In fact, clinical guidelines for treating depression published in the *Journal of Affective Disorders* now recommend 30 minutes of moderate-intensity exercise at least three times a week as a first-line treatment (graduated from second-line treatment in the past) for the mild-to-moderate depression so often seen in adults living with chronic illness.[15]

When a study from Duke University Medical Center randomly assigned female participants to either take drugs or do supervised physical exercise as treatment for mild-to-moderate depression, researchers found surprising results. The study's authors concluded, "This research suggests that both women taking antidepressant medications and women who exercise regularly can experience equal relief from their depressive symptoms."[16]

Karen Salmansohn, founder of the blog *Not Salmon* and author of *The Bounce Back Book*, shares something that has worked for her during her own darkest moments. She likes to ask herself this question, "What can I do right here, right now to feel better right here, right now?" She writes:

As the Buddhists say, "The 1,000-mile journey begins with one step." When you feel depressed about the chaos around you, simply breathe and focus on one small, easy action you can do in the short term. Repeat the following mantra: "I have it within me right now to get me to where I want to be later." This helps to give me a bifocal lens to view my life. It means you focus on both your short term and long term vision.[17]

The Stigma of Mental Health Problems

The word *stigma* means a negative judgment based on a specific personal trait—in this case, by a diagnosis of a psychological condition such as depression. The stigma of living with any form of mental illness diagnosis is pervasive in our culture, largely based on ignorance. In my own case, I had little if any personal experience with clinical depression, and—worse—I had little tolerance or comprehension of what it meant in others.

Here's an embarrassing example. I have a friend who has a friend who's been depressed, off and on, for years. During that time, my friend and I often wondered aloud why her friend couldn't just pull up her socks and quit all that self-absorbed moping around. We had no clue what we were talking about, but that didn't deter us from passing judgment on people who were too weak or too unmotivated to cheer themselves up.

Fast-forward several years to those weeks and months following my own heart attack. I knew something was very wrong with me. I could barely function. On some level, I must have suspected that what I was going through was something called depression. But I'm not the kind of person who gets depressed! That happens to other people—those weak, unmotivated people—but not to people like me.

I believed that myth because I was so ignorant about depression.

A study reported in the *British Journal of Cardiology* followed hundreds of heart patients for two years, of whom at least half showed symptoms of anxiety or depression when first interviewed. But the study authors noticed a common trait among this group. "Many of these heart patients seemed reluctant to accept a diagnosis of depression or anxiety, and expressed reservations to the clinical psychologist by rejecting the term depression to describe their problems, or by expressing negative views about attending a mental health service for treatment."[18] In fact, the negative views associated with the stigma of mental illness were so pervasive that all of the study's planned interventions had to be provided to the heart patients as part of a scheduled Cardiac Rehabilitation exercise program—instead of at a mental health facility.

Some patients are so reluctant to admit depression symptoms that they may not even mention them directly to their physicians. In a study called "Suffering in Silence: Reasons for Not Disclosing Depression in Primary Care," researchers found that stigma was behind the two top reasons for patients not telling their doctors:

1. fear of being prescribed antidepressant drugs
2. fear of being referred to a psychiatrist[19]

These fears are probably unique to mental health disorders. Can you imagine keeping the truth about a back injury or a migraine from your family doctor? There is no stigma surrounding seeking help for almost all physical conditions. But how is needing help for an acute psychological injury so different?

Sometimes people suffering from severely debilitating depressive symptoms—those who could likely benefit most from taking antidepressant medications—may even consider taking these meds to be a sign of weakness. Of course this is not true, just as it would never be considered weak for a person diagnosed with type 1 diabetes to take insulin. And remember that people struggling with depression are not able to control their moods, any more than people living with diabetes can use willpower to improve their blood sugar levels.

When I started doing my public presentations about women's heart health, I rarely if ever mentioned my own post–heart attack depression. Although I would briefly cover my story of misdiagnosis and survival, I figured that I had so much other important content I'd learned at Mayo Clinic to get through that I didn't have time to mention much else. And on some level, I know I felt hesitant to share such a personal disclosure from my past. I was unwittingly helping to perpetuate the stigma of mental health issues in heart patients by refusing to talk openly about my own.

But I changed my mind a few years ago. An audience member, herself a heart patient, raised her hand and asked me during one of my talks if I had experienced post–heart attack depression like she had been suffering. Nobody attending any of my presentations until that moment had asked me that direct question. I began answering her question, but was surprised by how choked up I began to feel, simply recalling how awful it had been for me. Even though it had been years since I'd been in the worst of those dark moments, that question was still a surprisingly powerful reminder of a devastating period.

But the interesting thing about honestly answering that woman's question was the feedback from other audience members following my talk. For days afterward, women contacted me to specifically thank me for speaking openly about the subject of post-cardiac depression; several said that before they'd attended that talk, they'd assumed they must be the only ones feeling that way.

I realized after that day that if I'm not willing to talk and write about my own experience of depression as a new heart patient, how can I expect others to do the same? If I let my own and society's discomfort with this subject stop me from sharing my own experience, how is that stigma going to be broken down over time?

When celebrities open up about their experience with depression or other mental health issues, it can often help the rest of us realize that these diagnoses are equal-opportunity realities. Rich or poor, old or young—mental health problems can strike any and all. When celebrities speak, it can break down unrealistic stereotypes about the sort of people who are diagnosed with mental illness. Canadian athlete Clara Hughes, for example, is a six-time Olympic medalist and the first Olympian in history to win multiple medals in both the Summer Games (cycling) and Winter Games (speed skating). After more than a decade of dominating athletic competition, she began to realize that her physical extremes were masking a severe depression. For a while, Clara tried to cope on her own with worsening symptoms, as she revealed in a *Toronto Star* interview in 2013. She fixated on trying to maintain her strenuous training regimen, and didn't even tell her mother what she was going through. The outwardly bright and engaging athlete felt isolated, began to gain weight, and cried every day. "I didn't know what it was. Nobody talked about it. Nobody talked about being depressed."[20]

She finally sought professional help after a national team doctor found her weeping in an airport. With the support of friends and family, her focus shifted to improving her health. Clara went on to win several more Olympic medals for Canada before her retirement in 2012. She now covers international sporting events as a sports broadcaster, and continues to raise awareness and support for mental health issues.

My plea to all physicians is now this: Doctors, next time you're seeing a freshly diagnosed heart patient for a follow-up appointment, please remember that we're more than just a major organ that's successfully undergone a cardiac procedure. It's time to start paying attention to the real-life emotional, mental, and psychological trauma embodied in the whole person sitting across from you. You want patients to follow your advice to take their meds, quit smoking, eat better, and exercise every day, and it's important to acknowledge that if they struggle with depression, their chances of doing all or any of those things will plummet.

I feel a bit embarrassed now, looking back at my profound pre–heart attack ignorance of mental health issues in general, and depression following a cardiac event specifically. Had I known more about how common situational depression actually is for heart patients, perhaps I wouldn't have suffered needlessly for as long as I did before seeking help.

6 ♡ I'm What a Person with an Invisible Illness Looks Like

Once a week, I show up bright and early for my Toastmasters club meeting, just as I have been doing every Thursday morning, year after year, since 1987 (when I was just a tiny baby). I love going to Toastmasters where, as our club guidelines promise, we get to practice becoming better public speakers, listeners, and thinkers.

I've had to miss several meetings, of course, in the weeks since being hospitalized—an absence that, sadly, will lose me the coveted annual Rise and Shine Toastmasters Club Attendance Award to my perennial archrival, Jim Johnson. Jimmy shares my wry amusement at our common dream—namely, no longer to win public speaking competitions, but simply to win an award for showing up.

I long to feel well enough to get back to my Toastmasters friends again. It's all part of this overwhelming need to somehow return to normal during a time when nothing feels normal anymore. It takes me several weeks, but I'm truly happy to be finally able to go back.

Precisely because early morning is now my best time of day (meaning minimal cardiac symptoms compared to the rest of the day), if you meet me for the first time at a Toastmasters meeting starting at 7:00 a.m. sharp, you will probably not be able to guess that I live with cardiovascular disease, including dreadful new symptoms of coronary microvascular disease (MVD). I look and sound remarkably like I used to, pre–cardiac event. I'm guessing that's why one of my fellow Toastmasters members comes up to me after my return to our meetings to ask me, "So, Carolyn. This is real, then? Not just, like—stress leave?"

No, you simpleton, I long to spit out at him. It's not just, like—stress leave.

But in fact, few people would be able to tell just by looking at me that I now live with significant heart disease, or that even the smallest outing with family or friends takes every bit of stamina I can muster, or that I need to nap like a preschooler every day just to manage the new normal that has become my life.

Few people out there realize how merely an hour or so of normal, pleasant conversation with friends over coffee can reduce me to a weak, shaky, frazzled heap by the end of our visit because of the sheer effort required. But I am a frazzled heap with a happy-face smile pasted on, of course.

Few people out there know how living with ongoing bouts of MVD symptoms like frightening chest pain, shortness of breath, or crushing exhaustion often requires a full day of physical recovery after each flare-up. It feels something like knowing you'll be knocked flat by the flu every other day, week in and week out.

And people don't see this because I look and sound pretty much the way I've always looked and sounded. When people tell me, "You look great!," what they don't hear is my inside voice silently shouting back, "If you only knew!"

But You Don't Look Sick

Most of us living with a chronic and progressive illness wake up, shower, brush our teeth, get dressed—and then go about our day, looking very much how we've always looked to the outside world. But to focus on just the outward-facing smile is to dismiss the reality of what life behind a facade of invisible illness can often be like.

Christine Miserandino echoes this observation on her popular website called *But You Don't Look Sick,* where you can read her powerful personal essay called "The Spoon Theory."[1] In this story of a coffee-shop visit with her friend, a handful of teaspoons is used to represent to the friend the limited daily reserves of energy (spoons) that must be carefully planned and counted out to get her through any average uneventful day as a patient living with a debilitating chronic illness. In Christine's case, her diagnosis is lupus, but she could well be speaking for all patients.

Her unique theory helps to explain what can be quite difficult to understand if you're healthy: how utterly exhausting it can be to get through even the simplest of tasks during a tough day of symptoms. Though facing a painful chronic condition since the age of 15, Christine has heard, from both well-wishers and physicians alike, "But you don't look sick," as if this annoying assessment were even relevant.

Worse, the words can somehow diminish and invalidate reality, implying that she can't possibly be as ill as she claims, given how good she looks at first glance. It's the curse of all who live with an invisible illness diagnosis—and a cruel irony at that, given that a curse is the last thing that sick people need on top of everything else.

A few years before I became a heart patient, I had a cycling accident while biking to work in downtown traffic. This accident resulted in a fractured bone in my foot (and the fastest land speed record in urban commuting history when I leaped instinctively from my face-down post-impact position in the middle of Wharf Street right up onto the sidewalk to avoid being flattened by oncoming traffic). I was in a bright purple knee-high cast for almost four months after that. I found it absolutely remarkable how solicitous perfect strangers became whenever they saw me coming, sporting my cast and crutches. I could clear the front half of my bus in five seconds flat every morning just by hobbling onboard. Considerate strangers would scramble to their feet in frenzied gallantry to offer me their seats. The irony was that I wasn't feeling at all sick. I felt terrific. I was able to work, travel, go to parties, and do just about anything I wanted to do except for driving (and biking, of course).

But many people who really do feel sick remain invisible to their fellow bus passengers unless they are using a clearly obvious assistive device. It's not that we want to look bad or draw attention to our medical conditions. Many of us, in fact, will go to great lengths to gamely keep up appearances in public just to maintain the illusion that we're doing fine, just fine.

I recall a woman in one of my heart health presentation audiences telling me after the talk that she felt "so much better now" about heart disease. "I used to be afraid of getting heart disease. But now that I see you here today—a heart attack survivor, walking, talking, looking perfectly fine—well, I'm no longer worried anymore!"

What? Remind me to go easy on the mascara and blush at my next talk.

In fact, I often do look "perfectly fine" even on those days when distressing cardiac symptoms are draining the life right out of me. On those days, I sometimes wish I could sport a leg cast or a neck brace or some other visible outward sign that something's not quite right.

It's important to keep in mind that there are invisible signs all around us, worn around the necks of people who are hurting—but we just can't read them. This is why I love the quote variously attributed to either Plato, Philo of Alexandria, or the children's author Wendy Mass: "Be kind, for everyone you meet is fighting a battle you know nothing about."

And if you've been fortunate enough to live this long with what's known as healthy privilege, it can be almost impossible to know anything about what living with an invisible illness is like.

Do You Suffer from Healthy Privilege?

I'd never heard about the concept of healthy privilege until I went to Palo Alto, California, in 2012, yet I'd been writing for some time about my niggling frustration over something that I didn't even realize had an actual name.

It all started when I met a whack of young (healthy! fit! hip! not sick!) Silicon Valley types while I attended Stanford University's annual Medicine X conference, thanks to being awarded an ePatient scholarship grant. Many of these young people at the conference seemed very busy designing, developing, and securing venture capital funding for their health technology startup companies that were creating tech magic like flashing/beeping digital pillboxes to remind us to take our meds each day. No matter what their magical game-changer, each one assured me that their invention was soon to become the Next Big Thing in medical technology, destined to change the world of health care forever (after which point, they would sell their startups to Google, retire as multimillionaires, and go surfing).

The more of these young tech types I met at Stanford, the more nig-gling my frustration became, mostly because the hype around their self-tracking digital miracles didn't seem to have Real Live Patients like me in mind.

It struck me that the imaginary patient meant to use their excit-ing new technology wasn't anything like me, or my *Heart Sisters* blog readers, or the women in my heart health presentation audiences on any given day. Had these tech guys ever been within a mile of an actual Real Live Patient?

Instead, the patient that the young hypemeisters talked about seemed to be some kind of fairy tale fantasy patient: tech savvy, highly moti-vated, compliant, eager to track every possible health indicator 24/7 on the latest apps, and most of all—oh, did I mention?—not sick. Their target market appeared in fact to be what we call the worried well, and not actual patients at all.

It turns out that there's a name for this attitude, and that name is *healthy privilege.* I was gobsmacked to learn this from Dr. Ann Becker-Schutte. She's a counseling psychologist in Kansas City who explained the concept like this on her eponymous blog:

> Many physical health conditions and all mental health condi-tions fall into the category of invisible illness. That means some-one who is casually looking at you might not be able to see the level of pain you experience. And they probably don't under-stand the effort that goes into a normal day.
>
> They don't see or understand because they have some degree of what I am calling healthy privilege. Healthy people enjoy the privilege of bodies that work in the ways that they expect, free from regular pain or suffering, without extraordinary effort. Healthy privilege allows healthy people to assume that their experience is normal, and to be unaware that coping strategies that work for them will not work for someone dealing with illness.[2]

Dr. Becker-Schutte was describing those young techies in Silicon Valley. But she could also be describing healthy family members, healthy friends, healthy work colleagues, or healthy care providers who may be well meaning but just don't get it, because they have always been so damned healthy.

What this means in everyday life is that there's a big fat difference between a highly engaged community that enthusiastically uses technology to track daily indicators such as weight / mood / motivation / sex life / food / exercise / bowel habits / hobbies / sleep / keyboard strokes (yes, seriously)—and actual sick people. And real people living with a debilitating chronic illness every day may lack the energy, ability, or will to commit to technology in any kind of meaningful fashion.

Or as Toronto patient advocate Kathy Kastner, author of *Death Kills, and Other Things I've Learned on the Internet,* mused one day on Twitter: "Self-tracking means you're focused on your illness all the time. Is data the answer to everything?"[3]

No, Kathy. More data is definitely not the answer to everything. Please pass that memo on to the Silicon Valley hypemeisters.

As a person living with chronic illness, I'm already feeling worn out most days from needing to focus on symptoms. My idea of self-tracking is putting a sparkly reward sticker on my bathroom cabinet calendar for each day I'm able to exercise. I used to award myself a sticker only for major physical accomplishments, such as an hour's brisk walk or an hour in the gym at Friday's weight-training class.

But unlike the keen followers of the Quantified Self movement (who seem to believe that if they didn't track it, it somehow didn't happen), I decided to change my unofficial reward policy recently to now include even the slowest of walks or the lightest of weights on a bad day. Feeling sick or in pain but still able to somehow talk myself into doing something, anything, other than what I really want to (which is to stay in bed with the covers pulled over my head) can feel like a real accomplishment. In fact, I believe that accomplishments like these are far more deserving of a sparkly sticker than anything I can do on a good day when I'm feeling well.

But sometimes, it's all just too much. Coping with a chronic illness is work. The work of being a patient includes managing medications, self-monitoring, visits to the doctor, lab tests, and figuring out how to incorporate important lifestyle changes into every single day. Did you know, for example, that a person living with type 2 diabetes could spend an average of two hours every single day, simply following doctors' recommendations for just that one condition?[4] Coping with all of those tasks requires time, effort, and cognitive work from both patients and their caregivers. And it is relentless 24/7 work that never takes a holiday. All of this can feel so overwhelming that being expected to embrace even one more additional task (like that self-tracking) can feel unbearable.

This is what Dr. Victor Montori, Professor of Medicine at Mayo Clinic, describes as "the burden of treatment" for patients with one or more chronic illness.[5] I'm very encouraged by his Mayo-based team's work on the innovative concept called minimally disruptive medicine. Patients not only must live with the burden of symptoms, but also with the burden of treatment provided by our health care system, as he explains:

> One of the key aspects of Minimally Disruptive Medicine is the need to become aware of the burden that our treatments cause on people's lives, to start thinking of the patient as being exposed to a workload, and having the capacity to do that work. We consider the workload involved in being a patient—and at the same time in being human, being a parent, a spouse, a worker, a teacher, a coach. But all of these roles compete for the same capacity.
>
> A patient's education level, literacy, state of depression, pain, fatigue, social connectivity and supports, financial status—all of these affect a patient's capacity to do the work. The workload can simply exceed the capacity to cope.[6]

Dr. Montori's team at Mayo's KER (Knowledge and Evaluation Research) Unit has even come up with a simple clinical tool called ICAN to help their medical colleagues minimize this burden of treatment for patients. ICAN (which means Instrument for Patient Capacity Assessment) focuses on a doctor's most essential question: "What's best for this particular patient?"[7]

But even the need for something like minimally disruptive medicine might seem head-scratchingly foreign to those living with the luxury that healthy privilege provides. One of the reasons that learning about the concept of healthy privilege had such a profound impact on me was that, until 2008 when I survived that heart attack, I had been fairly bursting with an insufferably smug sense of healthy privilege myself.

I knew nothing about what it might be like to live with a debilitating illness every day—and why would I? I'd been a distance runner for 19 years. I was a busy, active, healthy, happy person with many family, community, career, and social events penciled into a bulging calendar. And even though I worked in hospice palliative care for many years—and so saw firsthand countless patients and families dealing with end-stage disease—observing an ill person in bed means nothing in terms of understanding what illness actually feels like.

What I've learned since developing my own cardiac issues is that, until you or somebody you care about are personally affected by a life-altering diagnosis, it's almost impossible to really get what being sick every day actually means. Such is the bliss—and the ignorance—of healthy privilege.

"You Look Great!," and Other Things Not to Say to the Freshly Diagnosed

"Wow! You look great! You look just the same!"

In the early days post–heart attack, that was a fairly typical greeting from those who had not seen me for a while. While some might assume that this is a thoughtful, even flattering, comment to offer a heart patient, it often did not feel that way. Many women, especially in the early days, weeks, and months while still reeling emotionally and physically from their train wreck of a health crisis, report that they often feel like replying to such greetings with: "I don't feel great, and I am not the same!"

So, what might be more helpful to the freshly diagnosed than the well-meaning but oddly niggling "You look great!"?

"I'm Fine, Just Fine!"

Most of us are understandably reluctant to burden those we love by adding another layer of worry to their worries. We want to safeguard them from any undue anxiety our own health issues may cause them. I rarely if ever, for example, mention my symptoms to anybody except my physicians. I may have to sometimes change or postpone social plans depending on a symptom flare, but seldom ever feel the need to explain unless it's really, really serious (e.g., if I'm on my way to the hospital). It's ironic, isn't it? I may tire of having an invisible illness diagnosis, yet I try hard to keep it as invisible as possible to others.

But I know people who do feel this need to focus on reviewing each and every ache, twinge, or doctor's visit every time you ask them how they are, and I'm practicing how to not turn into one of them by remembering these positive ideas:

♥ You are not required to share personal details about your health just because other people ask.

♥ You're allowed to write whatever you like, and as much as you like, no holds barred, on any subject, especially your current health crisis, in a journal. Especially when you're feeling confused, angry, or overwhelmed, the act of journaling your deepest thoughts and feelings can often provide a unique perspective you may not have thought about before.

♥ You are allowed to pick and choose carefully which people in your life you decide you can trust when you do need to vent in person.

♥ You are allowed—indeed, encouraged—to feel truly blessed if you have somebody close to you who is a compassionate listener with a willing shoulder to cry on. Just try not to overstay the cry.

♥ You are also encouraged to take advantage of the in-person, virtual, or online WomenHeart support groups for women with heart disease[8] to ask questions or share what you're going through with others who really get it. It's free to join.

First, the urge to say something comforting and encouraging to somebody recovering from any serious condition seems like an instinctively kind-hearted gesture. My *Heart Sisters* blog readers, however, tell me that they suspect these comments more often reflect the relieved feelings of the speaker rather than the fabulousness of the patient's actual appearance. Friends and family alike can feel apprehensive that we might still look quite sick or different, and that this dreadful appearance might make them feel uncomfortable just being around us. Will it be awkward? Will they know what to say to us? How will they react if we look or sound really bad, if we don't look the same?

It's a similar reaction observed in end-of-life care by those of us who have worked in the field. Bereaved people are told by well-meaning friends and relatives, for example, in particularly chirpy tones, how great they look—this after the death of somebody they love. It can be hard to know just how to respond to such an irrelevant assessment of something as trivial as appearance when you are grieving. Most people simply try to be gracious, smile gamely, and say, "Thank you."

Like most of you, I've experienced my fair share of garden variety pain over the years (caused, in my case, by things like a ruptured appendix, broken bones, knee surgery, and popping out two babies the old-fashioned way). But none of those even came close to the chronic pain of *refractory angina* caused by my current diagnosis of coronary microvascular disease (MVD). The chest pain caused by this chronic disorder of the heart's smallest blood vessels is episodic, intense, and as frightening as my debilitating heart attack symptoms were—except that this kind of pain happens almost every day. And unlike headache pain or back pain, which can't usually kill you no matter how much it hurts, we're exquisitely aware that cardiac pain can. My pain can be mostly managed by medications (including my trusty nitro spray) as well as the non-drug, non-invasive TENS therapy recommended by both my cardiologist and my pain specialist at our regional pain clinic.[9] But severe chest pain flares (several times a week, sometimes several times a day) have essentially become routine for me.

And yet I apparently look the same, flare or not. I'm aware that, especially when I'm out in public, I tend to maintain this pasted-on little happy-face smile in order to keep up a pleasant facade of normalcy, and to avoid drawing attention to myself. When others see me now, walking, talking, sounding much like my old self, it can seem natural for them to make a comment about how I look (perhaps because of all this dopey smiling?). But they may not realize that, when you feel like hell, there's not much comfort in believing that you'll leave a good-looking corpse.

So, next time you approach a heart patient, a bereaved person grieving a loss, or anybody suffering with a chronic and progressive illness, what could you say instead of focusing on their outward appearance? One of the most helpful comments to me so far has been some variation of the simple greeting, "It's good to see you!" This is probably fairly accurate, feels pretty darned good to hear, and won't elicit the "If you only knew . . ." reply that we may be silently muttering.

Is Fake Smiling Unhealthy?

Speaking of pasted-on smiles, the classic song called "Smile" was originally written as an instrumental by the legendary Charlie Chaplin for his 1936 movie *Modern Times*. The catchy lyrics about smiling though your heart is breaking were added later, and the song became a hit for Nat King Cole in 1954.

But Nat's musical advice about faking a smile may be exactly the wrong thing to do for our own emotional health. This warning is particularly important for those living with a chronic diagnosis like heart disease, who often report feeling obliged to put on a happy face around others—even when feeling ill or frightened about their symptoms.

Many of my readers tell me that they often feel compelled to pretend to be fine so as not to worry their families or friends—even when they are quite clearly not feeling fine. They may even attempt to hide symptoms from their own physicians—as illustrated in the story from Leslea Steffel-Dennis in chapter 2.[10]

An astute physician I've known for a long time once said to me that keeping up a false front like this could be an occupational hazard after my 35-plus years working in the public relations field. In the wonderful world of PR, it doesn't matter if you have morning sickness or a migraine, you get to be remarkably skilled at attaching that big smile before tap dancing out to organize a fundraising gala, to deliver an after-dinner speech, or to facilitate a press conference for your clients.

But you don't need 35-plus years in PR to be an expert at fake smiles. I suspect that most people living with an invisible illness engage in pretend smiling on a regular basis. But according to authors of a study published in the *Journal of Personality and Social Psychology*, we do this at our peril: "Positive emotional behavior that does not accurately signal a person's experience—such as a smile that is not felt—may impede social connectedness and, in turn, psychological functioning."[11] (By the way, I could have told those researchers all about impeded social connectedness based on my 20 years of mind-numbing dinner party conversations trapped, along with my girlfriends, all of us still gamely smiling, between our scientist husbands going on all evening about zinc and copper sediment in the Fraser River estuary.)

These study authors suggest that smiling when you really don't feel like smiling is a form of dissociation that can actually predict poor health outcomes. Dissociation is the way our human psyche copes with intolerable circumstances, almost like a temporary escape route to help us survive.

Another interesting study on this phenomenon examined the differences between the effects of both our fake smiles and our genuine smiles. Researchers tracked men and women whose jobs require them to be courteous and endure frequent interactions with many other people all day long, day after day. They examined what happened when these subjects engaged in one of two behaviors: either surface acting (a fake smile) or its opposite, deep acting (an authentic smile generated through focusing on positive thoughts). The study found that on days when their smiles were forced, the subjects' moods deteriorated and they tended to withdraw from work, emotionally exhausted. These fake smiles are also known as emotional labor, meaning the suppression of feelings to provide a welcoming outward appearance. Ironically, trying to suppress negative thoughts may have actually made those thoughts even more persistent. (Please remember that fact the next time you're tempted to politely wear that fake smile while your dinner companions are droning on about shop talk, because the effect of negative thoughts was found to be especially significant in women.)[12]

Although the pretend smiles of surface acting may help to make other people around us feel comfortable, when these smiles don't genuinely represent how we feel inside, they may actually be hurting us. And when chronically ill patients exhibit this emotional labor on an ongoing basis (meaning that they feel one way, but act another so as to hide how they're feeling around other people), impaired physical health can result.

According to Michigan State University's Dr. Brent Scott, the study's lead author, women are both expected to and do show greater emotional intensity and emotional expressiveness than men. For example, "Women were harmed more by surface acting, meaning their mood worsened even more than the men and they withdrew more from work. But they were helped more by deep acting, meaning their mood improved more and they withdrew less."[13]

If those conclusions are not enough to make you want to start spending more time laughing at cute cat videos online, consider that fostering a genuinely positive outlook can particularly benefit those who are at significant risk for heart disease. According to a Johns Hopkins University study published in the *American Journal of Cardiology*, people who had a strong family history of heart disease and a cheerful outlook were one-third less likely to develop cardiovascular disease than their counterparts with exactly the same risk factor but who were not cheerful.[14]

Fake smiles, no matter how noble our motivation to practice them, are neither good for us nor for those unfortunate dinner party monopolizers, who are now mistakenly convinced, thanks to our enraptured surface acting, that they are not boring after all. But cultivating genuine smiles based on deliberate mood-enhancing strategies turns out to be very good for us indeed.

7 ♡ One-Downmanship: You Think *You* Have Pain?

Eventually, as the weeks and months go by and the symptoms of my acute heart attack crisis morph into even worse symptoms of the new cardiac diagnosis of coronary microvascular disease, I realize that I'm beginning to bore myself with my own exhausting story.

This is especially true given that I haven't died yet, and might eventually have to come to terms with this new reality. So one day, I try delivering this tough-love internal pep talk:

Yes, you have heart disease. Join the club.

Yes, you have pain and shortness of breath and overpowering fatigue. Get in line.

Yes, you don't want this to be happening to you. Well, it is.

Yes, that ER doctor who misdiagnosed you was wrong, the system is inefficient, and nobody understands you. Cry me a river.

Yes, you're confused and frightened and unsure about what's going to come next. Welcome to the human condition.

My self-absorbed bleakness doesn't entirely disappear after the tough-love lecture. Much of this need to obsess over my own story simply comes from somehow trying to make sense out of it all. But I'm beginning to believe that my little self-lecture might be starting to work whenever I'm compelled to interrupt somebody else's story, but decide that I don't need to.

I also catch myself pausing after other people casually ask me how I'm doing. I now wonder before responding if this is an appropriate person to share what's really going on for me today, or will a "Fine, thanks" do for now? (It almost always does, in fact.) And really, do I even have the energy, knowing by now that, for some people, the question "How are you?" is merely the minimal formality required before being able to launch into their own story? Or can I restrict my personal health updates to close friends and family members who honestly care and do want to know more?

At a cardiac rehabilitation class, the man next to me leans over and asks, "What are you in for?" I start to tell him that I've had what doctors call the widow maker heart attack, and that I had a stainless steel stent implanted, and . . .

He interrupts me to announce enthusiastically, "I have three stents!"

He then embarks on a blow-by-blow account, exquisitely detailed, about his cardiac event. I begin to feel that my own seems puny by comparison. Three stents? How can I possibly compete with that? My previously fascinating heart attack misdiagnosis story now seems hardly worth mentioning.

It strikes me that there are two things going on here. First, it turns out that there's some sort of competitive tension around the determination of who has suffered the most. (You think you have pain? Let me tell you about pain . . .) And secondly, many of us seem to have a pervasive urge to talk and talk and then keep on talking about our health problems. Attention must be paid!

Haven't We Earned the Right to Complain?

During the 19 years I spent as a distance runner, my running group (whose motto was: "No pace too slow, no course too short!") implemented a useful rule. The first ten minutes of every training run were devoted to whining. "My quads hurt. I'm so tired. I hate hills. I think I'm getting another blister . . ." But at precisely the ten-minute mark, our rule was: No More Whining. Let's face it—nobody is that interested. Just shut up and run, already.

For most people, the urge to complain about assorted health issues is understandable. Dave, my Santa Barbara friend, likes to call this the organ recital. But keeping up a negative running commentary about one's own health at the slightest prompt can become an entrenched habit if we get too good at it. This habit is especially seductive among those of us living with one or more chronic illness diagnoses, including heart disease. That's because surviving a heart attack or any other cardiac event can be such an overwhelming experience. Scary symptoms are truly awful. We worry about future dangers, and we want to rehash the horrible thing that's just happened to us. And haven't patients legitimately earned the right to keep telling their family and friends about what has happened, what is happening today, and what might happen tomorrow?

Talking about our physical complaints may make us feel temporarily better, but it may also hurt us in the long run, says Nova Scotia's Dr. Barbara Keddy, author of *Women and Fibromyalgia: Living with an Invisible Dis-ease*. Dr. Keddy has lived with fibromyalgia for five decades, and is also a heart attack survivor. On her blog, she describes a support group of Toronto women with fibromyalgia who get together regularly, but not, like virtually all other disease-specific support groups, to discuss their shared illness with each other. This group's ground rules: we talk about wellness only. As Dr. Keddy explains: "Reliving past injuries of a physical or emotional nature can reactivate the nervous system. Instead, it is more important to recognize our reactions, rather than the specific events related to the trauma."[1]

Dr. Keddy is not the only academic suggesting that the urge to whine may actually be hurting us. This self-focused ruminating can actually worsen physical symptoms. It's like relentlessly picking away at a rough scab, which then refuses to heal. Some patients can remain emotionally wounded for years by reliving and re-experiencing those distressing moments again and again.[2] But we also know that many other survivors can recover fairly well with the help of support or appropriate professional help.

When Yale University professor Dr. Susan Nolen-Hoeksema spoke about her rumination research at an American Psychological Association (APA) conference, she echoed Dr. Keddy's warning about the inherent dangers of such ruminating:

When people—especially women—ruminate about problems, they remember more negative things that have happened to them in the past, they interpret situations in their current lives more negatively, and they are more hopeless about the future. Ruminating can become the fast track to feeling helpless by paralyzing problem-solving skills. You can become so preoccupied with your problems that you're unable to push past the cycle of negative thoughts.[3]

She also warned that ruminating has a chilling effect on the willingness of others to put up with us. Friends and family members might respond to our ruminations compassionately at first when the health crisis is shiny and new, but this compassion starts to wear thin the longer we keep talking about the crisis. That's why ruminators report reaching out for others' help more often than non-ruminators do, but ironically, they actually end up receiving less of it, as Dr. Nolen-Hoeksema explained to her APA audience:

> Many ruminators report more social friction—things like people telling them to buck up and get on with their lives. After a while, others become frustrated and even hostile, and start pulling away, which of course gives ruminators a whole lot more to ruminate about, like: "Why are they abandoning me? Why are they being so critical of me?"[4]

Women exhibit a unique response to severe stress (such as a serious health crisis). Instead of what we know as the *fight-or-flight response* that's common in men, a cascade of brain chemicals in women are more likely to cause what researchers call a *tend-and-befriend response* to stress. This biochemical response actually drives women toward tending their children and gathering with other women for support during a crisis. It may also help to explain why women so often like to talk things out—even when talking and talking and talking appears to encourage unhealthy rumination.[5]

I'm not suggesting, of course, that the freshly diagnosed heart patient can't have the occasional meltdown that all of us are entitled to now and then. Instead, I'm talking about drowning in the deliciously seductive but unhealthy (and annoying) worldview that says, "All life sucks, but especially everything about my life. And now let me tell you all about it." Such self-absorbed focus carries the whiff of one-upmanship. One-upmanship compels us to do or say something in order to prove that we're better, smarter, or more interesting than others (as perhaps best displayed in that unfortunate 2013 hipster trend of sporting Google Glass on one's face in public).

Bragging about how bad you've had it actually looks like a competition called one-downmanship. You can tell if you might be engaging in one-downmanship if you have ever interrupted somebody telling you about their _____ (insert diagnosis / symptoms / medical procedure here) in order to:

♥ interject your own far more fascinating personal experience
♥ share a better story of another person you once met or read about in the tabloids or dated back in high school
♥ tell her about your own relatively minor health experience that's neither serious nor remotely relevant to the topic
♥ attempt to convince her to try the all-natural homeopathic gluten-free organic vegan herbal supplement you just learned about from a celebrity TV doctor (you know, those miracle cures that our physicians don't want us to know about)
♥ advise her that, clearly, her physician is _____ (insert the appropriate slur: in bed with Big Pharma / uninformed / greedy / an idiot), which then reminds you of something your own physician has said or done, which you can now commence describing to her at length

Finally, if you realize simply by reading this list that you seem to have a tendency to keep interrupting others no matter what they're talking about, please shut up and listen, for God's sake. And a gentle reminder that empathetic conversation is not merely waiting for the other person to take a breath so we can interrupt.

My Unspoken (yet Weirdly True) Hierarchy of Heart Disease

I came to observe during the weeks and months following my cardiac rehabilitation classes that many of us heart patients, consciously or not,

You Do Have the Right to Remain Silent

If you, as I did, ever get to the point where you're starting to bore yourself by telling and re-telling your own cardiac story to anybody polite enough to listen, Yale University's Dr. Susan Nolen-Hoeksema suggests these two key steps to help us minimize the urge to keep up that unhealthy ruminating on our medical woes:

1. *Engage in activities that foster positive thoughts.* "You need to engage in activities that can fill your mind with other thoughts, preferably positive ones," she recommends. That could be anything from a favorite physical activity to a hobby or meditation. (Personally, I use my grandchild, Everly Rose, as the best distraction ever.) The most important thing, says Dr. Nolen-Hoeksema, is to get your mind off your ruminations for a time so they die out and don't retain a grip on your mind.

2. *Problem-solve.* People who ruminate not only replay situations in their head, they also focus on abstract questions such as, "Why do these things happen to me?" or "What's wrong with me that I can't cope?" Try instead to identify at least one concrete thing you could do. For instance, if you just can't stop thinking about a confusing comment your doctor has made to you, commit to calling your doctor for clarification.[6]

seem to slot ourselves arbitrarily into what I now call the unspoken (but weirdly true) Hierarchy of Heart Disease. That man in cardiac rehab who interrupted my answer as soon as he recognized that he deserved more points than I did was offering a perfect example of how my Hierarchy works.

Herein I offer my unofficial and highly subjective personal rankings in the Hierarchy. If any of these cardiology terms seem foreign to you, check out my patient-friendly, jargon-free glossary at the end of this book. This will help you translate many confusing words and abbreviations. And by the way, I think I made this Hierarchy up. It's not in any medical textbook you'll ever find:

1. *Heart transplant* is the undisputed winner in the heart disease sweepstakes. Anybody who's survived a heart transplant (or is on the transplant waiting list) has experienced something so profound that, even among other organ transplant cases, no medical procedure beats this one. If you ever meet a heart transplant survivor, do not under any circumstance mention a lesser medical condition you may have. Trust me on this one. When there's a heart transplant in the building, nobody cares about you.

2. *Coronary artery bypass graft surgery (CABG,* or what we affectionately call *"cabbage").* This is major open heart surgery, sometimes under emergency conditions, that may or may not be associated with an imminent heart attack. Extra points if your CABG was preceded by an actual heart attack. This procedure is similar to a detour on the highway when there's a roadblock, except here blood vessels from elsewhere in the body are harvested to form new grafts in order to reroute the blood flow around blocked coronary arteries. Multi-vessel heart disease (affecting more than just one of the heart's major arteries) is more often seen in men; women are more likely to have single-vessel disease.[7] When it comes to CABG on our unofficial Hierarchy, more is better. Triple bypass tops double, quintuple beats quadruple. You get the picture.

3. *Heart valve repair or replacement* can require major surgery and, running neck and neck with CABG, often means having your sternum cracked open to get to your heart's faulty aortic, tricuspid, or mitral valves. You earn extra points if you have more than one valve involved. Deduct a point if you've avoided the carcass-cracking by having minimally invasive or keyhole closed-chest surgery.

4. *Blocked plumbing* means that a coronary artery is significantly blocked and may need to be opened up (revascularized) to help restore blood flow to the heart muscle, but not necessarily through major surgery such as CABG. An intervention to revascularize the heart may possibly prevent a heart attack if you haven't already had one by the time you make it to the hospital. Solutions can include invasive balloon angioplasty (inflating a tiny balloon

inside the blocked artery to smoosh the plaque), atherectomy (using a tiny Roto Rooter–type burr to grind the plaque into tiny bits), or a laser catheter (vaporizing the plaque).

Add one extra point if a stainless steel stent is implanted into the artery during an angioplasty procedure, unless this is an elective (non-emergency) procedure scheduled well into the future. But just as with CABG, the more stents, the higher your score. The *Journal of the American College of Cardiology* has actually reported the extraordinary case of a 56-year-old patient with 67 implanted stents, a kind of full metal jacket on steroids and the all-time winner in our stent sweepstakes, although the interventional cardiologist involved might be justifiably accused of showing off. Even researchers who have studied this case were compelled to ask, "How much is too much?"[8] Two bonus points if your stents were implanted as an emergency procedure because, like me, you were having a heart attack. Give yourself extra points if your heart attack was due to a spontaneous coronary artery dissection (SCAD),[9] a potentially deadly cause of heart attack usually seen in young, apparently healthy women with few if any cardiovascular risk factors.

5. *Electrical misfires* (or an arrhythmia) involve abnormal heartbeats, often requiring a device or surgical correction of some sort, such as a pacemaker, an ICD (implantable cardioverter defibrillator), cardiac ablation, or a cardioversion (cardioconversion) procedure. Heart failure (a truly unfortunate and scary choice of words for this common condition, formerly called congestive heart failure) is also sometimes treated with an implanted pacemaker or ICD. Add extra points if the arrhythmia involves serious inherited heart abnormalities such as Brugada syndrome or long QT syndrome that usually affect young healthy adults, or if sudden cardiac arrest preceded your diagnosis.

6. *Functional malfunctions* is the name I use for many other serious heart conditions such as cardiomyopathy (a number of different diseases of the heart muscle), endocarditis (infection of the heart lining or valves), myocarditis (inflammation of the heart muscle),

and pericarditis (inflammation of the outer membranes surrounding the heart)—all of which make it hard for us to function. Congenital heart defects are those present since birth, and they often lead to ongoing cardiac issues well into adulthood. There are now, in fact, more adults living with congenital heart defects than children because of lifesaving improvements in pediatric cardiology.[10] Heart failure, as mentioned above, is a dreadful name that needs to be changed (yesterday!) for a condition that affects heart function because the heart becomes less able to efficiently pump oxygen-rich blood to the rest of the body. The most dangerous loss of all heart function is sudden cardiac arrest. Quadruple points on the Hierarchy and a big high-five if you've survived that one.

7. *Drug therapy* by itself without the need for invasive cardiac procedures is used to nicely manage many types of heart disease. Examples include taking nitroglycerin for stable angina symptoms, and beta blockers, ACE inhibitors, calcium channel blockers, statins, blood thinners, or anti-platelet drugs for other heart issues. Check the glossary for more details on any of those terms.

8. *Other conditions.* I feel compelled at this point to add to my Hierarchy of Heart Disease the coronary artery spasm condition called Prinzmetal's variant angina.[11] You deserve double points if you have Prinzmetal's, mostly because its spasm symptoms are debilitatingly painful and often seen in younger women. Ditto for my own current diagnosis of inoperable coronary microvascular disease (MVD) that affects the tiniest of our tiny coronary arteries—too small to stent, too small to bypass, but equally debilitating.[12] Now if an actual heart attack (myocardial infarction) has preceded anything on this list, score an extra two points.

But before you pull out your own scorecard, remember that this is not and never should be a competition. Triple bypass surgery doesn't give you the right to lord it over a double bypass patient. This is one of the reasons, in fact, that I believe there's no such thing as a small heart attack, although many physicians seem happy to toss that descriptor around when trying to reassure new patients.

Even if a physician tells you that your cardiac diagnosis is relatively minor in the grand scheme of things, it may not feel minor at all. Such reassurance can miss the boat when it comes to acknowledging the profound psychological impact of surviving any cardiac event—no matter how much or how little heart muscle damage has occurred, no matter how successful medical interventions have been or not, and no matter how much others try to minimize mental health outcomes.

There Is No Fair Fairy in Life

In the year 2000, I started working in the field of hospice palliative care. That career experience was more educational than any university course I've ever taken, any book I've ever read, or any professional development training I've shelled out cash for. And the biggest lesson I learned over those years in end-of-life care stemmed from one simple truism:

There is no Fair Fairy in life.

In end-of-life care, we see unfair things happening day in and day out. Pretty soon, we learn that life is indeed not fair. Full stop. End of discussion.

I was reminded every day just how true this was when, for example, we had a 19-year-old admitted to our inpatient unit, dying of ovarian cancer. Or a mother in her early thirties leaving two toddlers and a distraught young husband behind. Or when we watched parents of any age grieving the death of their child, because we all know that it's just not right for parents to outlive their children.

Yet in the ongoing day-to-day drama that is Real Life—for those of us diagnosed with a chronic and progressive illness like heart disease, for example—we often want to wail about the unfairness of it all. In the early days post-diagnosis, I used to sometimes feel like an outraged toddler comparing the larger size of my sister's piece of cake with my own:

Why me?

I don't deserve this!

Why did this have to happen?

Many of us need to discover the secret of being able to move from wailing to acceptance, when what we really want to do is whine about the inherent unfairness of our plight.

Here's how Dr. Edward Creagan at Mayo Clinic shares his take on this issue. He warns us that there are at least three fundamental truths that cannot be ignored if we really want to move forward toward any semblance of serenity and well-being in life, no matter what horrible health crises have struck us en route. These fundamentals include:

> *Life is not fair.* The good people do not always win. And sometimes the best intentions are misguided or misinterpreted. Recognize your limitations—and those of others—and then move forward as best you can.
>
> *You are responsible for your actions.* Sure, you can complain. You can be critical, but at the end of the day, the buck stops with you.
>
> *The past is over.* The future is not yet here. So today—this moment, this place in time—is all there is. If you continually focus on the rearview mirror of life, if you take your eyes off the road ahead, chances are slim that you will safely reach your destination.[13]

Here's another tip: embracing attitude shifts like these must be a self-imposed act. They're not something you can shove into the faces of other people by waving in front of them a copy of Dr. Creagan's handy list of fundamentals.

When life has pummeled us into the peat, we also need time, self-compassion and perspective (along with those early bouts of weeping, wailing, and feeling very, very sorry for ourselves) until we finally feel ready to stop blaming that Fair Fairy.

Sometimes, life stinks. And yes, that's just not fair.

Looking for Meaning in a Meaningless Diagnosis

♥ Everything always works out in the end. (No, it doesn't. Things often get much worse, in fact, and sometimes never do get better.)

♥ This was meant to be. (No. It wasn't.)

♥ Life doesn't give you anything you can't handle. (A ridiculous claim. Life delivers truly horrific, unbearable outcomes all the time.)

My own general translation of such platitudes: "Blah blah blah . . . "
Here's one I like better: "Sometimes, bad things happen to good people."

It is often tempting to offer bumper sticker platitudes designed to somehow make people feel better about those bad things. We may feel that we have to say something comforting, and when we open our mouths, trite platitudes fall out. Nowhere is this effort to force people to feel better more pronounced than in the concept called Post-Traumatic Growth. We could define this simply as believing another platitude: what doesn't kill you makes you stronger. Or we could look at this slightly more complex definition: "Post-Traumatic Growth is the experience of positive change that occurs as a result of the struggle with highly challenging life crises. Although the term is new, the idea that great good can come from great suffering is ancient."[14]

It may be an ancient idea, but there are lots of ancient ideas I'm not buying any more than I'm buying this one. Surviving a catastrophic diagnosis doesn't make us heroic, any more than dying from that same diagnosis means we weren't heroic enough. For those who do embrace this concept, it's like saying that life before a health crisis was somehow meaningless, or that true meaning in life can only come after suitable degrees of suffering. We even use combat terminology to describe the heroine's journey, like the war on cancer, or battling heart disease, or exclaiming "She's a real fighter!"

So far, very little of my life since being diagnosed has felt to me like much of a battle. Mine is not a particularly heroic response against a chronic and progressive illness—unless you count simply getting out of bed in the morning. That's not much of a heroine's journey. My current diagnosis means I live with a uniquely painful and debilitating condition, but I'd never describe my daily response to it as any kind of heroism.

Society's emphasis on the need for brave positivity, even in the face of suffering, can wreak havoc on an already anxious sick person's struggle to seek meaning from distressing symptoms. For such a patient, a recurrence of illness or a decline in one's medical condition can feel like a personal failure born of a bad attitude, instead of what it actually is: merely the known trajectory of a given disease.

The implication of personal failure may be based on the not-so-subtle expectation that good patients will take the lemons that life pitches at us and make deliciously noble lemonade. What makes the triumph even more noble, especially for all those motivational speakers out there, are near-death health crises. The more traumatic the struggle to survive, the better the winning recovery lesson.

"Your illness has been a blessing in disguise!" The late Dr. Jessie Gruman said that she'd been told that many times by those who were impressed with her accomplishments as a longtime patient activist. She was, by every external measure, an iconic and beloved role model of how a patient can make lemonade out of lemons. Diagnosed with four catastrophic cancer-related illnesses and a dangerous heart condition, hers was an international reputation, earned as president and founder of the Center for Advancing Health—a nonpartisan, Washington-based research institute that she ran from 1992 until her death in 2014. Dr. Gruman was the author of six books on patient engagement, and the recipient of nine honorary doctorates in recognition of her dedication to improving the patient experience. But in a compelling essay on her website, she questioned the validity of that "blessing in disguise" theory.

> The belief is that sickness ennobles us, that there is good to be found in the experience of illness, or that while diseases are bad, they teach life lessons that are good. But this common belief about the nature of suffering from illness is inaccurate, and can inadvertently hurt sick people and those who love them.
>
> If I do not find spiritual or philosophical benefit from my illness, I fall short: either I haven't tried hard enough or I'm not smart enough to do so.[15]

Dr. Gruman argued that illness is no different from any other life event: sometimes we learn from experience, and sometimes not. Conceding the argument that, within the adversity of illness, she'd somehow "found the calling and the commitment to speak out on behalf of people who are ill," she immediately added that this was neither a sign of her virtue nor of her will: "I would trade that commitment in one hot second to not have been sick in the first place."[16]

My concern with this Post-Traumatic Growth expectation for patients is that not only are we supposed to survive a health crisis, but we'd better do this recuperation thing right so that we can emerge triumphantly at the other end with a suitably life-enhancing meaning that points us (and other people) toward a shiny new future.

This existential search for meaning in illness appears to be pervasive throughout medicine, says author and political activist Barbara Ehrenreich, writing in the *Guardian* about her breast cancer diagnosis in 2010.

> The first thing I discovered is that not everyone views the disease with horror and dread. Instead, the appropriate attitude is upbeat and even eagerly acquisitive. The more fellow victims I discovered, the greater my sense of isolation grew. No one among the bloggers and book writers seemed to share my sense of outrage over the disease and the available treatments.
>
> In the mainstream of breast cancer culture, there is very little anger, no mention of possible environmental causes, and few comments about the fact that, in all but the more advanced metastasized cases, it is the treatments, not the disease, that cause the immediate illness and pain.[17]

Barbara's experience led her to confront the puzzling concept of illness as a gift. As she described to her *Guardian* readers, a serious diagnosis is often viewed as "not a problem at all, not even an annoyance. It is a gift, deserving of the most heartfelt gratitude."

I agree with breast cancer blogger Nancy Stordahl, author of both the aptly named memoir *Cancer Was Not a Gift and It Didn't Make Me a Better Person* and her award-winning blog *Nancy's Point*, when she explained:

> It's impossible for me to be grateful to a disease that killed my mother in a very slow and painful manner. It's impossible for

me to be grateful to a disease that has killed dear friends of mine and others I care about, knowing countless more struggle every day in unimaginable ways. And it's impossible for me to be grateful to a disease that might yet swallow me up as well. It's unfathomable for me to be grateful in any way, shape or form.[18]

I can, with enough practice and determination, learn to adjust, to cope, to manage, to function, to put one foot in front of the other in order to adapt to this new normal of living with ongoing cardiac issues every day, but please don't insult me by implying that my diagnosis was somehow a lovely gift-wrapped present that I must have needed in order to bring meaning into an otherwise meaningless existence.

I also understand writer Kevin Drum's perspective on his own diagnosis of multiple myeloma, an incurable form of blood plasma cancer, as he described in *Mother Jones*:

I sometimes wonder if I'm the only person in the world who hasn't learned a deep life lesson. I haven't battled it. I've just done the stuff my doctor has told me to do. I haven't become more aware of the fragility of life. I always knew about that. I have cancer, and even I get tired of the virtually endless parade of "brave" movie stars going on *Access Hollywood* to talk about their struggles.[19]

When a serious medical crisis strikes, it by definition becomes the central focus of life. Everything else is now of lesser importance in this forced march toward first surviving and then normalizing a new reality, to try to get back to where, who, and what we were before we became patients. Perhaps this is why we feel the urge to keep talking about what's happened to us. We're just trying to figure this all out, seeking the elusive silver lining that we keep hearing about. Although, as Kevin Drum also observed in his essay: "I don't mind talking about it. The reason I generally don't is because it makes other people uncomfortable."

Am I saying that maintaining a positive attitude isn't important? No, of course not, as we have just learned from that interesting research on surface versus deep acting reported in the last chapter.

By nature, I've always been a generally happy and optimistic person (and, as my sleepy family can attest, early morning is when I'm the most relentlessly cheerful). I like being around other positive people. And it appears that, optimistic or not, we all have untapped resources of resiliency that may never be needed until a crisis strikes. But when it does, we simply continue, getting up, showing up, and doing our best to make our way as foreigners in this new country.

If you insist on seeking meaning in bumper sticker platitudes, let's heed this wise Buddhist reminder, simply put: "Pain is certain; suffering is optional."

Inspiring versus Inspirational

I can't be alone in wondering why most inspirational speakers and writers do not inspire me. Call me cynical, but maybe I've heard once too often:

♥ Follow your dreams!
♥ Reach for the stars!
♥ Eat more kale!

These pep talks are typically delivered with varying degrees of cheerleading conviction by speakers who spend considerable time boasting about their own amazing dream-following, star-reaching, or kale-eating accomplishments. If anything, once the rosy glow of the hype wears off, I find these pep talks de-motivating, particularly on a day when I'm already feeling worn down by chest pain, shortness of breath, or crushing fatigue. On those days, I might be able to admire the tenacity of people who are able to reach their goals in the same way I can admire the zeal of triathletes, measured by the volume and velocity of vomit at the finish line. But these role models more often leave me feeling weak and inadequate—not inspired at all.

Most inspirational speakers, I'm guessing, do start off sincerely trying to help their audiences by sharing what they genuinely believe will work for listeners in order to _____ (insert lofty goal here).

So here's my concern with the dreams/stars/kale inspiration model. As social scientists often point out, *inspirational* messages are simply about the intention to inspire, while truly *inspiring* messages demonstrate the effect of becoming inspired based on our internal reactions and outward actions in response to that message.[20]

Thus, an inspirational idea happens *to* you, while an inspiring idea happens *within* you. Inspiration involves both being inspired *by* something, but far more importantly, *acting on* that inspiring thing. Otherwise, based on results, it means that the inspiring message wasn't that inspiring after all, and that you have just wasted a whack of cash on yet another personal growth seminar.

This is a relevant topic for those of us living with chronic illness. Our dedicated health care providers are always trying to think up better ways to somehow inspire the freshly diagnosed patient to:

♥ take these pills
♥ eat this food
♥ quit those cigarettes
♥ do these exercises
♥ monitor those test numbers
♥ manage that stress
♥ keep those medical appointments
♥ stop doing that
♥ start doing this

Yet the sad reality is that no matter how demonstrably sound the advice, most of these inspirational messages remain remarkably unsuccessful in actually inspiring patients to be more compliant (a distasteful and patronizing word to many patients, by the way, that sounds like it has punishment at the end of it).

The World Health Organization estimates that, for a variety of reasons (none of which include the need for a flashing/beeping pillbox), barely half of all patients actually take their medications as prescribed.[21] And a Canadian study that investigated 7,500 people living with cardiovascular disease in 17 countries found that, despite their doctor's orders,

▼ 18 percent continued to smoke
▼ 65 percent did no exercise
▼ over 60 percent did not adopt a heart-healthy diet[22]

Not being able to inspire people to achieve these health goals is a significant problem in medicine. Ironically, it has always been so, as the ancient Greek physician and teacher Hippocrates wrote back in the fourth century B.C. "Keep a watch on the faults of the patients, which often make them lie about the taking of things prescribed. For through not taking disagreeable drinks, purgative or other, they sometimes die. What they have done never results in a confession, but the blame is thrown upon the physician."[23]

What inspires you to start or stop behaving as your physician recommends may be quite different from what inspires me to take action. Here, for example, is a simple message that I personally found inspiring. It's from the late US tennis legend Arthur Ashe, and it's focused on other people, not on his own stellar accomplishments or those of other elite athletes like him. His words made sense to me as a person trying to enhance my own ability to influence my life as it is now, every day, one small step at a time—especially on days when I'm feeling really ill. Best of all, I think it's applicable to many other goals or challenges.

The Ashe message is this: "Start where you are. Use what you have. Do what you can."[24]

But I Don't Want to Be a Patient Anymore

There's a peculiar tendency among those of us with a chronic and progressive illness diagnosis that I believe is underappreciated by our health care providers. It's the profound need to just be a person, and not a patient anymore.

How many times have I wished in vain for precisely this? How often do any of the recently diagnosed tire of debilitating symptoms and meds and fear and exhaustion and hospitalizations and treatments and medical appointments and tests and more tests? How tempting it is to dream nostalgically about life as it used to be, before we became patients. Remember when you were just a person, and not a patient?

In the movie version of this fantasy, the dark clouds would part, rays of morning sunshine would kiss the curtains and cardiac meds lined up in the bathroom cabinet would miraculously evaporate while a harp played glorious background music, and we would all awaken from this nightmare about the day we became patients. But this isn't a movie, and I've never been able to undo my diagnosis with just positive thinking or creative wishcraft.

I met a man one day in my cardiac rehabilitation group who had recently passed the one-year anniversary of his quadruple bypass open heart surgery. He confided to me that he had recently decided to stop taking all of his heart meds. On top of that, he had started smoking again. I remember looking at him as if he had just sprouted two heads. "Why don't you just jump off a cliff and get it over with?" I wanted to shout at him about these suicide-on-the-installment-plan choices.

It turns out that my cardiac rehab friend is not alone. There are many cardiac survivors who seem to view their doctor's orders like they do New Year's resolutions: a flurry of panic-fueled determination at first, followed by hit-and-miss efforts, followed by quitting.

While our medical providers are working hard to make sure that we follow instructions they believe will help us stay healthy, live longer, or even avoid recurring crises, they're often working with a group of people who want our old lives back, thank you very much, and who simply do not want to be patients any longer. That sentiment may well be the key to understanding the differences in health care goals between the physician offering the best of care and the patient who too often seems to be rejecting that offer.

This is particularly problematic in chronic care, which in terms of human history, of course, is a relatively new concept. A century ago, our average lifespan was about 50 years. Our ancestors tended to die from acute health crises involving infections, epidemics, childbirth complications, or devastating industrial accidents. Far fewer people lived long enough then to develop the chronic illnesses we face today.

We all know that following our doctors' orders is clearly expected if we're trying to be good patients. Not doing what our doctors recommend seems just plain crazy, doesn't it? Consider the question of why patients don't take important medications as prescribed by physicians. Some commonly held theories include:

♥ cost (some doctors may not ask if expensive meds are affordable)
♥ distressing side effects (which may not be taken seriously even when reported)
♥ the challenge of managing multiple prescriptions (take those three pills once a day, this one twice a day, and these two three times a day)
♥ cultural issues (some studies report that factors like lower socio-economic status and language barriers can significantly impact patient behavior)[25]
♥ forgetfulness (sometimes responsible for a patient's non-intentional behavior)
♥ uncertainty about the actual need for the meds (if the drug relieves pain, we'll probably take it; everything else, not so much)
♥ anxiety and depression (can have an effect on a patient's ability to follow basic discharge instructions about physical activities, smoking cessation, and taking meds as prescribed)
♥ the burden of treatment, as discussed in chapter 6 (often sums up all of the above)

And maybe, as doubtful as this possibility might seem to our physicians, patients don't do what they're told when those patients just want to be people again.

8 ♡ On Being a Good Patient

There are small moments of most days now, usually in the pre-dawn hours, still in bed before I even start stretching the kinks out of sprawled limbs, when I experience a strange waking dream. In this dream, I actually forget that I'm a heart patient. I forget about that heart attack, or that I still live with the ongoing symptoms of a serious cardiac condition. In these small moments, I feel good. Life is good. Early mornings are good. I am not a patient anymore.

But reminders to the contrary start quite soon after lifting myself out of that bed. I'm reminded that I have heart disease when I pour out the fistful of heart meds I must take every day, presorted every Sunday evening into my colorful days-of-the-week pill box that lives on the lower shelf of the bathroom cabinet.

I'm reminded again whenever I have to book yet another medical appointment with my family doctor, my pain specialist, or my cardiologist. Medical appointments. Waiting rooms. Diagnostic tests. Hospital procedures. More waiting rooms.

Yet even though I seem to spend more time around health care providers than I ever imagined I'd be doing, the reality is that I'm the one who deals with virtually every day-to-day cardiac issue on my own. Each year, I spend hours following up with my physicians, but I spend 365 days trying to manage my symptoms myself. As one of my *Heart Sisters* blog readers astutely said to her own cardiologist: "This is your career, but it's my life."

I'm reminded whenever I unpack my little black TENS unit box. Every morning, I clip the small device onto my belt, or tuck it into a hip pocket, and then very carefully attach its sticky electrode pads onto the skin around my heart, tucking their long black wires under my clothes. I adjust two tiny knobs on my black box to the correct power levels and feel a prickly little buzz pulsating across my chest. Prescribed by my cardiologist, and followed up on regularly by the pain specialist at our hospital's regional pain clinic (who—luckily for me!—spent a year doing a cardiology fellowship in Sweden studying the refractory angina of microvascular disease), TENS therapy is far more familiar to cardiologists overseas than it appears to be here in North America so far. As the UK National Refractory Angina Centre confirms, "Neuromodulation should be offered as part of a multidisciplinary angina management program based on current guidelines."[1]

I'm reminded whenever I refer to my wonderful cardiologist as *my* cardiologist. I still don't think of myself as the kind of person who needs to have her own cardiologist.

I'm also reminded that I have heart disease, oddly enough, during those little moments when I'm feeling pretty good, when I'm in between symptom flares, when I feel happy and alert and—Oh! What's this? No pain?—when I'm appreciating how deliciously blue the sky is or how heartbreakingly sweet my little granddaughter Everly Rose's voice sounds. It can seem that these moments can flit away almost as soon as they begin, so I've learned to love them even more before they do.

Everything I now know about heart disease, I've learned and continue to learn since having my own. Mostly, I'm learning how little I knew back then, and how many smug preconceptions about chronic illness I embraced, thanks to my own healthy privilege. Being diagnosed with heart disease or with any other chronic and progressive condition has an impressive way of turning life upside down and shaking us until the smugness gradually starts to fall out.

How Acute Illness Compares with Chronic Illness

Here's how to be a good patient:

♥ Get sick with a short-term acute ailment.
♥ Get an appointment to see your doctor.

♥ Get diagnosed.

♥ Get a prescription.

♥ Get better.

♥ Thank your brilliant doctor.

Now, here's how to be a difficult patient:

♥ Contract a chronic and progressive illness.

♥ Go see your doctor.

♥ Get diagnosed.

♥ Take your meds.

♥ Get diagnosed with something different. Many, many times.

♥ Take your new meds.

♥ Keep going back, because symptoms keep getting worse.

♥ Get more tests.

♥ Take different meds.

♥ Get referrals to specialists. Many, many times.

♥ Get more tests, more meds, and more invasive medical procedures.

♥ Keep going back.

You get the picture . . .

That sums up the difference between diagnostic categories. You may have found yourself on the first list of those who have sought treatment defined as acute care medicine (broken bones, pregnancy, strep throat, ruptured appendix, knee surgery, etc.). Acute care medicine is a branch of secondary health care in which we receive active but short-term treatment for an injury, for an episode of illness, for an urgent medical condition, or during recovery from surgery. Acute care medicine is not the same as chronic care medicine, and thus patients being treated for acute care conditions are not at all the same as patients living with one or more chronic illness diagnoses, including heart disease.

Coincidentally, I've experienced each of those (temporary) conditions listed as acute care examples, which means I have at least some awareness about what it's like being on the receiving end of acute care. During each incident, I figured I knew what being a patient was all about, but under relatively short-term treatment. I knew nothing about how different that experience was compared to being diagnosed with a chronic illness.

Whenever an acute care episode is over, it's usually over for good. We become, quite simply, no longer patients. In fact, I propose that acute care is not, despite the insistence of the "we-are-all-patients" folks, what actually being a patient is about at all, as I discovered only after being told in 2008 that I have significant heart disease.

The pain and debilitation of being acutely ill usually gets better. The pain and debilitation of being chronically ill can last forever. In fact, many living with chronic illness feel terrible. Every. Single. Day. And while those receiving acute care can expect that the experience of feeling temporarily terrible will gradually diminish, in chronic care we often live with the chilling knowledge that it feels bad now, and it's likely to get even worse over time.

Are You Being a Difficult Patient?

When the Emergency nurse scolded me for having questioned her physician colleague about that odd pain down my left arm, the message I heard was clear: keep your mouth shut. My question had demonstrated to her and to that physician that I was being a difficult patient. She had to put me in my place.

Her stern little lecture, which I believe to be fortunately rare among health care providers (certainly among the nursing team I worked alongside for many years at the hospice), left me feeling embarrassed because I'd obviously been making a fuss about nothing, and also humiliated because I'd also apparently offended the doctor by asking a question. So when my cardiac symptoms inevitably returned, no wonder I felt reluctant to seek help from the same health care providers who had already labeled me as difficult.

You may have experienced your own variation of this reluctance. You arrive early for your doctor's appointment. You wait patiently, and when you're finally ushered into the exam room, you don't complain about having to wait. You try not to take up too much of the medical team's valuable time. You sit across from the doctor; you nod and smile politely during the visit. You pick up the prescription for your medication, thank the doctor, and walk out the door to make room for the next patient waiting.

And sometimes you do this even when the discussion about those meds or your overall health leaves you with unspoken concerns or unanswered questions. Many of you know what this feels like, so it may be reassuring to learn that academics are studying the pervasive fear among patients of being labeled as difficult.

Consider the research on this unique fear published in the journal *Health Affairs*. It focused on participants who had voiced a strong desire to engage in shared decision making about their treatment options with their physicians. The people recruited for this study were from Palo Alto Medical Foundation physician practices, described by the researchers as "wealthy, highly educated people from a desirable suburb in California, generally thought to be in a position of considerable social privilege and therefore more likely than others to be able to assert themselves."[2]

As residents of Silicon Valley, they also represented one of the most wired health populations on the planet. Participants in this study were generally over 50, living in affluent neighborhoods, and had either attended or completed graduate school. Yet here's how researchers explained their reality: "Most participants in the study talked about how they actively tried to avoid challenging their physicians during office visits. Deference to authority instead of genuine partnership appeared to be the participants' mode of working with physicians."

Researchers observed three obstacles that can inhibit patients' important interactions with their physicians, including:

1. Even relatively affluent and well-educated patients feel compelled to conform to socially sanctioned roles and defer to physicians during clinical consultations.
2. Physicians can be authoritarian.
3. The fear of being categorized as difficult prevents patients from participating more fully in their own health care.[3]

In my experience, my blog readers who worry about being perceived as difficult are often also afraid that the quality of their care might be affected. And they might be right to worry. In a 2016 study published in the *BMJ Quality and Safety* journal, researchers reported that doctors make more diagnostic errors when dealing with patients they label as "difficult" compared to their non-disruptive "neutral" patients.[4]

As Dr. Dominick Frosch, lead author of the *Health Affairs* study, explained in a *New York Times* interview in 2012:

> Many patients still aren't perceiving the relationship with their physician as a partnership. Yet patients should play a role because they live with the outcomes of care. People experience a different sense of self in the doctor-patient interaction. The clinical context creates a reluctance to be more assertive. And it's hard to think that people from more disadvantaged backgrounds would find it any easier to question doctors.[5]

I had the same observation when I read about his study. I was in Palo Alto when I attended Stanford University's Medicine X conference in 2012, and I have to ask: if even these "wealthy, highly educated people" feel compelled to defer to authority when communicating with their physicians for fear of appearing to be difficult patients, do the rest of us dull-witted average people have a hope in hell of not doing so, too?

It may seem disrespectful for doctors to label a patient as difficult, but make no mistake—there are indeed those people for whom "difficult" would be a charitably accurate descriptor; we've all met these pain-in-the-neck types in our travels. But my concern is for those patients who are generally reasonable, curious, and not-difficult—the people who simply want to ask a question (but may hesitate), or to discuss specific treatment options (but may hesitate), or to be taken seriously when feeling ill and desperate (but may lose hope of doing so) because of a profound reluctance to be unfairly labeled.

I've heard from a surprising number of my *Heart Sisters* blog readers who share alarming reports of being treated like difficult patients because they had originally challenged a doctor's dismissal of their cardiac symptoms. These patients can be maddeningly frustrating to health care professionals, because doctors may not be able to solve a diagnostic mystery or find a treatment option that works, and worse, they may dread encountering these patients again due to that frustration.

So patients like me walk a razor-sharp tightrope. We risk being labeled as difficult if we persist, yet we risk being dead if we don't.

And we are justifiably afraid, in case something is actually wrong, of being dismissed and sent away. No wonder many of us simply resort to "deference to authority" like those nice, well-behaved Palo Alto patients do, too. And no wonder study author Dr. Frosch made this plea: "We urgently need support of shared decision-making that is more than just rhetoric. It may take a little longer to talk through decisions and disagreements, but if we empower patients to make informed choices, we will all do much better in the long run."

So no matter how uncomfortable or scary it may feel at the time to be seen as difficult, all of us need to speak up, ask questions, and be our own best health advocates.

The Patient Voice

There are patients. And then there are patients.

Let's consider, for example, two friends of about the same age, same size, same socioeconomic demographic—each one (in an amazingly freakish coincidence) a survivor of a similarly severe heart attack, admitted to the same hospital on the same day. Let's call these two made-up examples Betty and Boop.

Betty's heart attack symptoms are taken seriously and she is diagnosed promptly, treated appropriately, recovers well, suffers very little if any lasting heart muscle damage, is referred by her well-informed cardiologist to a program of supervised cardiac rehabilitation, is surrounded by supportive family and friends, and is happily back at work and hosting Sunday dinners after a few short weeks of recuperation.

But Boop, on the other hand, experiences complications during her hospitalization and takes far longer than expected to recuperate. Her

Carolyn's Top 10 Tips on How Patients Should Be Treated

Dear doctors, nurses, and hospital staff,

Some suggestions on how kindness and courtesy can help your patients today:

1. Acknowledge the existence of patients by smiling, introducing yourself, and explaining the procedure/test you'll be doing for them today.
2. Make eye contact when you are speaking to another human being.
3. Don't make assumptions that patients know anything at all about the procedure that's about to happen just because you routinely do these same procedures day in and day out. Patients can feel distressed just thinking that there might be something (else) wrong with their hearts.
4. Remember to say something like, "Today's test/procedure will start with _____, and then we'll do _____, and then finish up with _____." Even for patients who already know what to expect, it's common courtesy to review this information for them.
5. Please don't use medical jargon to explain what you're about to do to your patient's body.
6. After the explanation, ask your patient, "Do you have any questions for me about today's procedure?" before you begin.
7. Be considerate of your patient's privacy and dignity. Stripping to the waist is not a big deal to most men, but it is a very big deal to women—especially with a man sitting in the same room who has not bothered to introduce himself. And by the way, next time I'm ordered to strip to the waist in front of a strange man, he'd better buy me dinner first.
8. Immediately offer your patients a private or curtained-off area to remove their clothing, a clean, folded hospital gown, and a surface to put their clothing on when ready, so they're not standing there half naked in a cold room, clutching

(continued)

sweater and underwear in front of strangers, and wondering what to do next.

9. Wash your hands. No patient should ever have to ask you to do this before you touch them.

10. Always try to imagine yourself in the shoes (or hospital booties) of every patient you see today, and consider how you would like to be treated, too.

Your patient,
Carolyn

cardiologist fails to refer her to cardiac rehab, she has little support at home from family, her cardiac symptoms worsen, expensive repeat hospital procedures are required, she suffers long-term debilitating consequences, and is never able to return to work.

Yet despite these profound differences, physicians would still describe both of these women with the same straightforward descriptor: myocardial infarction (heart attack).

The family, friends, neighbors, and co-workers of the freshly recovered Betty now think they know what a heart attack is like (based on their own personal observations of her). And given how Betty has bounced back, heart disease must not really be that bad after all. Her cardiac problems are fixed. Life is pretty much back to the way it's always been for her and for those around her. In fact, it's better, as Betty now realizes how precious life is and decides that from now on, she will live her life to the fullest!

Meanwhile, the family, friends, neighbors, and co-workers of Boop cannot quite figure out what's going on with her. They learn that having heart disease must be horrible. Boop seems to be still dragging her sorry ass around, not bouncing back like her friend Betty has already done, no longer acting like her old self, distressed over her worsening condition, worn down by ongoing cardiac symptoms, and very worried about her future. One day, Boop hears a cardiologist interviewed on a TV talk show who describes people like her as cardiac cripples, who might be fixable if only they would develop a more positive attitude. This makes her feel even more distressed and hopeless.

That TV doctor is not the only one making assessments like this. It's as tempting to define Betty as a good and admirable patient who's doing everything right as it is to accuse Boop of having somehow failed at being a good patient. We generally like hearing from positive people like Betty, and we feel uncomfortable listening to negative stories from those like Boop. Compared to her friend Betty, we might even judge Boop as no longer even trying to get better—because, like many people living with chronic illness, and as everybody around her agrees, she certainly looks perfectly fine.

So which is the more accurately representative heart patient example?

A trick question, dear readers. There is no such thing as a one-size-fits-all patient—no matter what the diagnosis happens to be, and no matter what medical textbooks tell us. This is precisely why you must never under any circumstances start entertaining the freshly diagnosed heart patient with irrelevant stories of your Auntie Marge and her heart attack. Nobody else is like Auntie Marge, and new heart patients simply do not care about her.

I often remind others of this: even though I'm a heart patient, a Mayo Clinic–trained patient activist, a writer, and a public speaker who has spoken to thousands of women about what I learned at Mayo about women's heart health (and more importantly, have also heard the voices of thousands of women through my blog), I can't possibly represent all heart patients when I write or speak. I can't claim to do this any more than one physician speaking onstage can pretend to speak for all other doctors.

This is why I'm always so glad to see more than one patient voice represented at health care conferences—happily, an increasingly frequent event often identified by Patients Included accreditation that acknowledges event organizers who deliberately include patients on the stage, in the audience, and at the microphone.[6] Similarly, full-time family caregivers, parents, or spouses of patients represent critically important voices, especially when more than one of them are invited to speak at the same event—yet this demographic is an often-overlooked resource.

Just recently, I told a conference room filled with health care administrators and bureaucrats that, while I was glad to accept their invitation to volunteer my personal perspective during their Patient-Centered Care planning meeting, all I could guarantee was that my views would be those of just one person. Me, and only me. I really wished there had been more than just me representing the patient voice that day. Otherwise, I often feel that I'm merely a token tick box to be checked off on some event planner's To Do list.

Common Courtesy in Medicine

I showed up recently for a scheduled (non-cardiac) medical test in the medical imaging department at the hospital. It was one of those particularly distasteful tests that involve a full day's prep at home, choking down a range of hideous chemical cocktails, consumption of which is designed to induce explosive liquid diarrhea that requires staying extremely close to a toilet all day long. The procedure itself on the following morning was right up there on the Creepy/Disgusting/Embarrassing/Cringe Scale of medical experiences.

Hospital procedures like this can feel invasive, distressing, and revoltingly undignified for most patients. All the more reason that medical staff need to start treating us like we're more than just the nameless, faceless ten o'clock appointment in Bed #8, or what I like to describe as the obstacle between them and their next coffee break—like a piece of meat on a slab, but worse, an invisible piece of meat.

Call me crazy, but I believe that patients deserve to be treated with common courtesy, and let's start with the simple basics of saying something like: "Hello. My name is ____ and I'll be doing your ____ today."

This courtesy was a key element of the powerful campaign for more compassion in health care launched by the late UK physician Dr. Kate

Granger, who was also a terminal cancer patient. She'd felt appalled by the lack of common courtesy she was observing from the other side of the gurney between the time of her diagnosis and her death five years later at age 34. As an example of how bad some of her patient experiences were, she liked to tell the story of the physician who broke the news to her that her cancer was incurable. He was unable to look at her, and "couldn't leave the room quickly enough," as described in her obituary in the *Guardian*.[7] Her compassion awareness campaign focused on encouraging all of her medical colleagues to simply introduce themselves by name to each patient. She coined the #HelloMyNameIs hashtag to help the idea spread around the globe.

In a March 29, 2014, response to my *Heart Sisters* blog post on this topic, Dr. Kate wrote to me: "I believe this is more than simple common courtesy. I think it is the beginning of a therapeutic relationship, building trust and a human connection in which you as the patient feel comfortable to share your fears and anxieties or to let intimidating examinations happen."[8]

Consider, by comparison, the young man who greeted me that morning in our hospital's medical imaging department. Well, perhaps greeted is not quite the right word . . .

Rather, he stood in the doorway of the large room where I lay clutching my drafty hospital gown, an IV already poked into place in my right arm. "So, you must be Carolyn?" he mumbled, reading from my chart without actually making any eye contact whatsoever. I replied: "Yes, I am. And who are you?"

He actually seemed surprised that I would attempt to engage him like this. But since surviving my heart attack, I have decided to stop meekly tolerating poor manners from health care providers. It's taken a cardiac event to arrive at this decision. I approach each situation with friendly politeness, of course, in order to avoid that pesky "difficult patient" label.

I'd worked in that same hospital for many years, by the way, so I can appreciate that underpaid and overworked staff can sometimes have a bad day. But I'm not talking about your average bad-day behavior. I'm talking about a pervasive trend that Dr. Kate Granger identified when she first became a patient. So here's how I mentally approach a scenario like that with this young man and others like him:

Carolyn's First Basic Rule of Interpersonal Healthcare Communication: "Do not under any circumstances let a man who hasn't bothered with the simple courtesy of introducing himself start sticking objects up your bum."

Exam Room Etiquette

Harvard University's Dr. Michael Kahn once wrote an important editorial in the *New England Journal of Medicine* about the need for his colleagues to demonstrate and model good manners (or what he termed "etiquette-based medicine") during their interactions with patients—even as he admitted at the time that the very notion of good manners in medicine might seem "quaint." As he explained:

> When I hear patients complain about doctors, their criticism often has nothing to do with not feeling understood or empathized with. Instead, they object that "he just stared at his computer screen" or "she never smiles" or "I had no idea who I was talking to." I believe that medical education and postgraduate training should place more emphasis on this aspect of the doctor-patient relationship—what I would call etiquette-based medicine. There have been many attempts to foster empathy, curiosity, and compassion in clinicians, but none that I know of to systematically teach good manners.[9]

Dr. Kahn came up with a staff checklist for health care providers for that all-important first meeting with every hospitalized patient in order to help improve patient-physician rapport:

1. Ask permission to enter the patient's room—then wait for an answer.
2. Introduce yourself, showing an ID badge.
3. Shake hands (wear glove if needed for infection control).
4. Sit down. Smile if appropriate.

5. Briefly explain your role on the medical team.
6. Ask the patient how he or she is feeling.

Aside from wondering why it's even necessary to have to tell an intelligent, educated person to smile, I thought that Dr. Kahn's list was a great model for etiquette-based medicine. The big question at the time, of course, was: would other hospital doctors embrace this approach?

Five years later in his follow-up study, Dr. Sean Tackett from Johns Hopkins University School of Medicine concluded that "etiquette-based medicine was infrequently practiced" among the doctors who were studied. In fact, Dr. Tackett's team found that the physicians he observed performed not one of Dr. Kahn's six recommended behaviors with almost a third of all new hospital patients. Physicians did not explain their role on the patient's medical team to over half of new patients. And what they were least likely to do was to express interest in learning how new patients were feeling about hospitalization or their illness (only 4 percent asked about this).[10]

In another study, researchers at Northwestern University in Chicago found that only one-third of the hospital patients they studied could correctly name even one of their hospital physicians. But here's a telling statistic: twice as many could correctly name all of their nurses.[11]

When Docs Become Patients, They Become Better Doctors

I've heard physicians say that it was their unexpected experience with their own serious illness that taught them what med school couldn't, namely, that being the one wearing the hospital booties actually helped to make them better, more compassionate, and more empathetic care providers for their patients.

One of the most compelling stories I've heard about was in an essay by Dr. Itzhak Brook about his own experience as a physician facing throat cancer. He gives this personal example of the profound helplessness and dependence that can so often accompany becoming a hospital patient:

On one occasion, I asked a senior resident to clean my obstructed tracheotomy tube. He reluctantly complied, but did it without using a sterile technique, and flushed the tube using tap water. The tube he wanted to place back was still dirty, and when I asked him to clean it better, he abrasively responded, "We call the shots here!" and left my room. I felt humiliated, helpless and angry at being treated in this fashion.[12]

Dr. Brook, a professor of pediatrics at Georgetown University School of Medicine and author of the book *My Voice: A Physician's Personal Experience with Throat Cancer*, believed that encountering awful experiences like this while he was a hospital patient made him far more sensitive to what his own patients and their family members were going through. As he later wrote:

> I now try to avoid the patterns of behaviors that were offending and distressing to me, and to be more compassionate and caring. I now strive to model myself in the same pattern of devotion, warmth and genuine care I felt from some of my caregivers. I know now better than before how critically important they are. I also realize that by doing that I set an example to the physicians in training and students I teach.[13]

The lessons learned by these doctors-turned-patients often represent the daily reality, over and over again, for those of us who live with a serious medical issue. No matter how experienced and no matter how naturally compassionate these doctors may be, their new awareness of personal patienthood can come as a shock when they truly comprehend firsthand what their patients have been describing to them all along. It's one thing to listen to others complaining about being demoralized, humiliated, and frightened as patients, but physicians really do get it when they're the ones feeling that way.

Welcome to our world, doctors.

Not that I would ever wish a catastrophic medical condition upon any human being, but just as Dr. Brook, the late Dr. Granger, and so many other health care professionals have been unfortunately forced to discover, becoming a patient can end up being a priceless form of education that so far has never been adequately taught in med school. If only they didn't have to get sick to finally learn it.

I'm Tired of Being a Good Patient!

As a heart attack survivor with an accordion file of ongoing complications, I've become a frequent visitor to my cardiologist, my family physician, related specialists, the Pain Clinic, our local hospital, and countless diagnostic labs. One such diagnostic procedure that investigates my heart function is called a stress echocardiogram (that's a two-for-one test special: part running on the treadmill with EKG leads attached, and part leaping off the treadmill periodically to lie down on a gurney for an ultrasound recording of the heart).

My last stress echo experience was so profoundly upsetting that I not only complained to the departmental manager at the hospital, but—at her request—I created for her staff a list of basic guidelines (that you'll find in the chapter sidebar) on how to act respectfully around a bunch of half-naked sick people. Incidentally, as a Canadian, I live in a nation that's resigned to our stereotype as uniquely polite and apologetic, so you can appreciate that lodging an official complaint was a fairly big deal around here.

I must add that it wasn't the specific diagnostic procedure itself that was so upsetting that day, but the appallingly poor social skills of the two attending technicians in the room. For example, when I entered the echo lab, one of the two techs present sat at a corner desk. He did not look up at me when I walked in, did not say hello, did not introduce himself. Was he the tech? Was he the doc? Was he the janitor? Who knew?

As I later wrote to the departmental manager, "It's not so much that these people were openly rude, but it was their insufferable lack of people skills that pushed me right over the edge. No introductions, no eye contact, no consideration of how awkward this test can be, no explanation of the test procedure or even the flimsiest effort at basic politeness."

As I also explained to the manager, I was already feeling worried about this stress echocardiogram when I first arrived at the echo lab that day. That's because there is no such thing as a routine test when you're a heart patient. You're there because something bad has happened to your heart, or because your doctor suspects that something bad might happen soon, or to find out if something bad is happening right now.

When I was finally told to strip to the waist by that tech in the corner, neither he nor his colleague offered me a place to change or to leave my clothing. So I slowly pulled off my sweater and bra and clutched them in front of me to cover up a bit while the two techs sat in bored silence, waiting for me to finish up. Eventually, one casually motioned to a chair in the far corner of the room for me to place my belongings, and tossed (yes, tossed) a paper gown toward me. Neither could have possibly demonstrated less respect, even if they had deliberately set out to humiliate me. They simply could not care less. In fact, it was that sense of dismissive detachment that first made me think, "Something is very wrong with you people!"

I've had many, many medical procedures, scopes, and tests (not to mention those two babies I popped out), but none left me feeling as vulnerable as I felt during and after that experience in the stress echo lab. Most health care professionals I've encountered who administer privacy-invading procedures for a living have been generally kind, considerate, approachable, careful to explain what was happening, and solicitous of how I was doing throughout. People who are not like that should never be employed in health care positions.

When I reread my "Top 10 Tips on How Patients Should Be Treated" list, I realize that I'm now a much different person. Back then, I was far too worried about not making a fuss or being difficult (the same personality trait, by the way, that kept me from returning to the ER, despite worsening cardiac symptoms). I was so concerned about being a good patient that I became too willing to passively ignore what it takes to be a good echo tech, or a good nurse, or a good doctor, or even a good person.

But I'm tired of being a good patient.

I'm tired of tolerating intolerable behaviors, tired of politely putting up with the kind of rudeness and indifference that, had my kids demonstrated it when they were little, would have earned them a big time-out and no bedtime story.

If this experience in the echo lab were happening today, I would not hesitate to speak directly to either of these men, asking them to leave the room while I got undressed, but not before they demonstrated a minimal shred of common courtesy by introducing themselves to me. But why should it even be necessary to ask intelligent, educated people to behave like this around a vulnerable population like patients?

Courtesy and good manners in medicine should not be too much to expect.

9 ♡ The New Normal

Some days, I feel a wee bit surprised that I'm still alive. I've experienced ongoing cardiac issues, more hospital tests, and more procedures since those long-ago first cardiac symptoms hit. My subsequent new and improved diagnosis of coronary microvascular disease has meant that I have had to leave the job I loved with the hospice society, and the colleagues I loved working with for so many years. I now restrict all activities happening late in the day due to episodes of chest pain, shortness of breath, and crushing fatigue that seem to worsen as the day goes by. And I've learned the delicate balance required in knowing when it's time to go home.

And yet I'm still here!

I've learned that anxiously ruminating about my heart health every day can often morph into a chronic and exhausting state of being hypervigilant, that surreal fear that something bad is just about to happen. Not only is hypervigilance not conducive to feeling happy, productive, or like my old self, but it can also be damaging to my chances of overall future health.

Yet perversely, even successfully surviving weeks, months, or years without dying as planned doesn't necessarily reassure me that death is not, after all, just around the corner. Staying alive in itself may just not be enough to push through each new sudden painful twinge that catches me off guard, making me wonder if I should call 911.

But very gradually, almost imperceptibly, month by month, I am starting to feel less hypervigilant. I am no longer as afraid as I once was that I'll die in my sleep tonight. I am no longer convinced that every significant bout of terrifying chest pain means that today is the day I will have another heart attack. (It might be today, but I just can't be absolutely sure anymore.) I now review those years since 2008 and ask myself: how many hours/days/weeks/months/years did I focus more on what might happen than on what actually happened?

I am no longer wary of settling into what some people like to call "the new normal." For a long time, I've tried to resist using that phrase, mostly because part of me, the crazy-out-of-touch-with-reality part, still wants to embrace the fantasy that I'll wake up tomorrow and maybe none of this will be true after all. And then my life will indeed be normal once again.

Facing these issues means that much of my life now seems divided into what I was able to do BHA, before heart attack, and then AHA, after heart attack. No matter how you slice it, the scope of my AHA list remains a much-diminished reality compared to that BHA list. That's because debilitating physical symptoms are not only significant, but almost always accompanied by emotional fallout—an under-appreciated and rarely acknowledged companion to most forms of chronic illness that can indeed make physical suffering feel far worse.

But at our hospital's regional pain clinic, I'm learning more about pain self-management. I'm also meeting many others living with pain far worse than mine, caused by a variety of conditions—a reality that seems to make me feel luckier than most. Not lucky to have sustained the cardiac issues I have, but lucky to be able to do more than they can.

It occurs to me now that this is how my life might actually be from here on in. Based on results so far, it's highly likely that I may never return to my pre–heart attack self. And I know that it's taken me a long time to arrive, skidding heel marks and all, at a realization that perhaps has been blindingly obvious all along. I can either choose to focus on all that I've lost, or I can focus instead on what I still have.

The Cure Myth

In a perfect world, our doctors embrace the concept of curing what ails us. Even in the face of incurable diagnoses, the pervasive dream of a cure can persist.

Here's how I look at this issue of cure. When I spent a month in the hospital around my sixteenth birthday following a ruptured appendix and a near-fatal case of peritonitis, I was very, very ill. The surgeon later told my worried parents that I was lucky to have survived at all. But from the moment I was finally discharged from the hospital (a green rubbery abdominal drainage tube still nicely attached through a partly open incision), I can honestly say that I never again worried about my recently departed appendix. I never needed to. My appendicitis and its associated deadly complications were cured.

That's acute medicine for you.

But heart disease is not an acute illness. It's chronic and it's progressive. And we know now that a significant risk factor for having a heart attack is having already had one. As explained in the British Heart Foundation's *Heart Matters* journal: "However much of your heart is affected, a heart attack means you have heart disease, which is usually incurable. All heart attacks come with a risk of long-term problems, such as abnormal heart rhythms and a higher risk of a second heart attack or stroke."[1]

Cardiologist Dr. Stephanie Moore of the Heart Failure and Cardiac Transplant Program at the Massachusetts General Hospital Heart Center confirms this reality in her video interview on her hospital's website. "One reason some women aren't too concerned about heart disease is they think it can be cured with surgery or an angioplasty procedure and they won't have to worry about it again. This is a myth! Heart disease is a lifelong condition and once you get it, you will always have it."[2]

Yet I met many women during my Mayo Clinic training at the WomenHeart Science and Leadership Symposium who clearly believed that, once successfully treated, their heart disease was cured and gone forever. Some of you heart patients reading this might also think that. You may believe that the lifesaving cardiac intervention that you had was, in fact, lifesaving. Evidence suggests, however, that the best your treatment procedure can do is to address your current cardiac symptoms—not the root problems that originally caused them, often decades earlier—and it won't prevent your death from a future heart attack.[3] Cardiac interventions typically address only one specific blockage in a specific coronary artery at a time, but not the coronary plaque or inflammation that's affecting other arteries, now or in the future.

In fact, you may be surprised to learn that our care model in treating the coronary artery disease that usually causes heart attacks is arguably built around opening blockages in patients with late-stage heart disease. These are treatments that may relieve immediate symptoms, but that's about it.[4] And as I now like to tell my women's heart health presentation audiences, I didn't have a heart attack because I ate a piece of bacon that morning, or had a stressful day at work. My heart attack was instead probably due to something that damaged those very delicate endothelial cells lining my coronary arteries years, even decades, ago.

I once had a conversation on Twitter with cardiologist Dr. John Erwin, who heads up the Texas chapter of the American College of Cardiology. We were pondering why it's far harder to convince heart patients, compared to cancer patients, to make healthy lifestyle improvements post-diagnosis. His response: "Patients who come into hospital with a heart attack, who get a minimally invasive stent procedure done and who feel great the next day are hard to convince that they haven't been cured."[5]

The issue here, of course, is that when doctors and patients use the word *cure*, they may mean quite different things. As a patient, I'd define cure as the moment I'm told that whatever damaged my precious coronary arteries (again, years before experiencing my first ever symptom) is now gone, never to threaten any other arteries. But in reality, the best treatment outcome I can hope for now is simply a kind of détente.

I remember clearly the day that this reality hit home for me. I was sitting in a large room at Mayo Clinic on the first evening of our five-day WomenHeart Science and Leadership training program. Each woman who had been accepted to attend this training was asked to stand and introduce herself to our group of 45 other heart patients. I heard first one, then another, and another and another repeat some version of "I had two stents implanted after my first heart attack in 2002, then one of my stents failed so I had to have open heart surgery in 2006, and then my next heart attack in 2008 . . ."

Wait a minute! Not me, I wanted to cry out. My heart attack was a one-time-only deal. It happened. It's over. I survived it. I'm done. I'm fixed. I'm never going through this ever again! But as I sat there, mesmerized yet scared by repeated tales of serial cardiac events, I slowly began to believe all that I'd been reading and hearing about heart disease being a chronic and progressive diagnosis.

While existing cardiac treatments certainly cannot promise to cure heart disease (despite the misplaced belief of many patients that they do), there is some encouraging news here. We now know that up to 80 percent of heart disease may be preventable in the first place by paying attention to some basic lifestyle issues:

♥ Focus on eating more heart-healthy foods (e.g., from the widely studied Mediterranean Diet[6]) and far fewer high-sugar or high-salt processed foods.

♥ Exercise, exercise, exercise—or, as Kentucky cardiologist Dr. John Mandrola recommends: "You only have to exercise on the days you plan to eat!"[7]

♥ Learn how to improve how you react to stress.

♥ Do more of what you love doing, and far less of what you don't.

♥ Develop healthy sleep habits.

♥ Quit smoking—all smoking.

♥ Monitor and/or keep your blood pressure, cholesterol, and/or blood sugar numbers within the targets you've discussed with your physician.

♥ Monitor your cardiac health indicators throughout pregnancy (a history of pregnancy complications such as preeclampsia or gestational diabetes is strongly linked with higher risk of future heart disease).[8]

♥ Take all of these risk factors seriously, especially if you have a family history of heart disease (mother or sister younger than age 65 at the time of her cardiac event, father or brother younger than 55).[9]

Addressing these factors is especially important for those of us who are already living with a cardiac diagnosis. Consider, for example, the groundbreaking research on the importance of physical exercise for heart patients done by Dr. Rainer Hambrecht of Bremen, Germany. His research team found that 90 percent of the heart patients he studied who rode bikes regularly (but had not had coronary stents implanted) were free of heart problems one year after they started their exercise regimen. But among similarly diagnosed heart patients who did get a stent (but without the first group's regular exercise routine), only 70 percent were problem-free after that year. As Dr. Hambrecht told his colleagues at the time: "It's difficult to convince people to exercise instead of having an angioplasty, but it works. But there are multiple forces working against a scenario in which regular exercise is prescribed. Patients, for example, are not motivated to take responsibility for improving their own cardiovascular health—even if it means better event-free survival."[10] Follow-up studies continue to support Dr. Hambrecht's findings. For example, another study in 2016 conducted by his colleague Dr. Sven Möbius-Winkler reported "a significant improvement" in coronary artery blood flow in heart patients who participate in regular moderate exercise.[11]

Taking steps to minimize our cardiac risk factors is completely up to us. No pills, no fad diet, no miracle vitamin supplement, no health guru, no celebrity physician on TV will do this for us. The truth is that there's just no shortcut to making small but important lifestyle improvements.

The reality remains that sometimes, we just don't know what causes people to develop the kinds of heart disease that they do. You can spend your life lying on the couch, chain smoking and eating Tim Hortons Maple Dips—yet never, ever have any issues with your heart. Or you can be like many of the women in our group of heart patients at Mayo Clinic, ages ranging from 31 to 71. Included in this group were triathletes, vegans, and even a healthy young physician who was the most surprised heart patient in the building. These women had done everything right, and yet still developed heart disease. As already pointed out in chapter 7, there is no Fair Fairy in life.

Profound Life Lessons from Heart Disease

As one of my *Heart Sisters* blog readers once wrote to me, "I have more balance in my life now—because I have to!" Please don't wait until you get sick to mull over these important lessons:

1. When in doubt, just take the next small step.
2. Be kind and generous to your family and friends.
3. However good or bad a situation is, it will change.
4. Today is special enough to burn the candles, use the good china, wear the fancy lingerie.
5. "NO!" is a complete sentence. Practice saying that.
6. Time does heal almost everything.
7. Don't take things so personally.
8. Get outside in the fresh air every day—Mother Nature is waiting there for you.
9. No matter how you feel, get up, dress up, and show up.
10. Never lose your sense of curiosity about the world and other people.

Learning to Love Your Open Heart Surgery Scar

Each scar on my body tells a story. The big long one that tracks across my lower right abdomen tells of that appendix rupture on my sixteenth birthday. Two scars on my right knee tell of surgery after an unfortunate slide down a pile of gravel. Another meandering zigzag tells of a nasty piece of broken glass once embedded into my left palm, its evidence exquisitely masked by the skilled plastic surgeon who sewed my hand back up.

Women who have undergone open heart surgery sometimes have traumatic stories to tell about their very noticeable chest scars, and varied responses about whether to hide or not to hide this evidence, particularly in the early weeks and months post-op when scars are most noticeable.

After I wrote an essay on my *Heart Sisters* blog about the impact of these surgical scars on female heart patients, the response was decidedly mixed. A 45-year-old woman told this story, for example:

> I had double bypass open heart surgery five months ago. I feel so sad about my scar. Sometimes I cry when I'm in the shower, or if I try to wear a shirt and can't wear it because it shows. I watch my friends at the pool wearing bathing suits while I'm sitting on the side watching them, wearing a t-shirt and shorts. I just don't want to be there. I wish I could remove my scar. I'm so stressed about it.[12]

But conversely, another reader proudly described her chest scars as "a map of illness and recovery." Another explained the unconventional strategy she employs in response to unwanted public attention her surgery scar sometimes attracts:

> A gentleman walked past me at a local Target. He was staring at my chest pretty intently. I ran into this guy at least another two times while shopping, with him walking towards me staring openly at my chest. I think he was trying to get a better look at the scar.
>
> "By the third time, I pointed directly at my scar and said to him: "Bear attack!"

The last word on scars goes to the heart patient who summed up her philosophy like this: "A scar is never ugly. We must see all scars as beauty. Because take it from me, a scar does not form on the dying. A scar means I survived!"

Practicing Resilience

One of my audience members described my public presentations on women's heart disease as "part cardiology boot camp, and part stand-up comedy!" As odd as it may seem to be laughing during a heart attack story, there is a surprising amount of laughter throughout my talks. In hindsight, both my audiences and I can laugh at my freakishly puzzling reluctance to return to the ER despite my worsening heart attack symptoms. Women laugh together in knowing familiarity because we've all been there, making everything else more important than we are.

I've noticed that frightening stories can often become funny in the re-telling as time passes. None seemed one bit amusing when they were actually happening, of course. But it turns out that being able to look back with amusement instead of horror may represent a stage of resilience, a turning point when you're trying to adapt to a health crisis.

Psychiatrist Dr. Steven Wolin told a *Psychology Today* interviewer that there are, on the other hand, elements of our culture that seem to glorify victimhood. As he explained: "There is a whole industry that would turn you into a victim by having you dwell on the traumas in your life." But for some of us caught in the midst of such struggle, even the thought of being resilient while suffering can seem like an impossibility. Dr. Wolin reminds us that it's harder to feel like a victim if you're willing to consider creating new ways of being.

> Even talking about resilience can make some people feel that no one is really appreciating exactly how much they have suffered. In reality, you have considerable capacity for strength, although you might not be wholly aware of it.
>
> Resilient people don't walk between the raindrops; they have scars to show for their experience. They struggle—but keep functioning anyway.[13]

Sometimes resilience can only be identified in hindsight. It took Jodi Jackson five years after surviving a massive heart attack before she was finally able to reflect accurately on her own resilience:

> As I was laying in the hospital five years ago, my world as I knew it imploded and I didn't think I'd actually live another five years. At the time, my diagnosis felt like a death sentence. I was only 42. How was this all possible? The mistake I made at the time was trying to look five years ahead, but not looking at today for today. But that was the way I was used to living— always living in the future and not stopping for today.

As I started to live one day at a time, heart disease became manageable. I did the things I needed to do to make sure I lived one more day, each day. Being a heart attack survivor defined me in the beginning, and that was a good thing. I took it, I spoke publicly on women and heart disease, I shared my story. I worked with Go Red for Women and the American Heart Association educating other women. It is important work and I spent a lot of time doing it. I developed friendships I will always have with other survivors of heart disease and stroke. I cherish those, and honestly can't imagine what my life would be like without them.

My five year anniversary makes me feel like I am going to live. I feel hopeful and feel like, although this is something that is still a part of my life, it isn't going to get me any time soon! With that feeling, I can look forward to growing older and celebrating each birthday.[14]

Social scientists also tell us that humor can improve resilience by providing a positive impact on recuperation. The known connections between our brains, our behaviors, and our immune systems apparently respond to laughter (in fact, even anticipating laughter can affect these connections). Studies also suggest that humor not only boosts our health-protecting hormones, but can also reduce our levels of potentially damaging stress hormones.[15]

Gallows humor is one thing that's helped patients through some of the darkest times imaginable. Such dark humor isn't escapist, nor does it deny the awfulness of adversity. For example, a woman who had survived sudden cardiac arrest (twice!) told me with a big laugh that she now chooses the clothes she'll wear each morning based on "which sweater I least mind the E.R. team cutting off with scissors."

One day, in a strangely giggly mood, I started a new discussion topic on WomenHeart's online support community forum for women living with heart disease that elicited hundreds of responses after I invited other heart patients to complete the sentence, "You know you have heart disease when . . ." Here are some of their humorous replies:

♥ your idea of matching lingerie is two hospital gowns so you can wear one backwards as a robe so your tushie isn't hanging out

♥ you're not sure if your phone's set on vibrate or you're in atrial fibrillation

♥ you know how to hook up your own 12-lead EKG—and then interpret the results

♥ people say, "You look good!" and they sound surprised

♥ you only know what day it is because that's what your pillbox tells you

♥ you have to tell the slightly alarmed aesthetician doing your pedicure not to panic at the Plavix/aspirin bleeding from your cuticles

♥ your husband asks if you want to run upstairs and make wild, passionate love—and you ask which one does he really want, because you can't do both

♥ your nitro spray sleeps next to you on your bedside cabinet

♥ people ask you, "Did you know you parked in a handicapped person's spot?"

♥ your daughter sends you flowers on your graduation day—from Cardiac Rehab

♥ you see a woman wearing a red dress pin, and you hug her[16]

Or consider as well this real-life dialogue, shared by the patient herself, between an Australian woman and a cardiologist in her hospital's Intensive Care Unit. She says she was too groggy to remember much of this conversation, but her hubby swears that it actually happened. She'd been admitted to the hospital with congestive heart failure and familial dilated cardiomyopathy; she was about to undergo surgery to have an ICD (an implantable defibrillator) inserted into her chest.

Cardiologist: "And what brought you to the hospital?"
Patient: "An ambulance."
Cardiologist: "No, why are you here?"
Patient: "Isn't this the Hilton?"
Cardiologist to another cardiologist: "We have a live one here!"
Patient: "Gosh, I hope so. Let's try and keep it that way."[17]

Working versus Not Working

When the dust settled after my heart attack, all I wanted to do was feel like my old self again. I was convinced that what would most help me to feel normal was just getting back to work. But because of ongoing cardiac symptoms caused by my as-yet undiagnosed coronary micro-vascular disease, it was almost three months before my doctors finally granted me medical clearance to return to my public relations job at the local hospice society, half-days only to start. Ironically, my work-place was in the same hospital that had discharged me just a few short months earlier. By then, I was feeling especially relieved to get back to work because I'd already used up all of my paid sick time and all of my vacation days. Symptoms or not, I knew that I simply could no lon-ger afford to stay home with no money coming in.

But after the first flush of welcoming hugs from my hospice col-leagues, it very quickly became apparent to me (and worse, to them) that I was just no longer able to function while juggling multiple dead-lines, all due yesterday—the normal hair-on-fire pace in the world of PR. I'd enjoyed a high-profile and successful public relations career for over three decades, and being forced into early retirement in my fifties hadn't ever been on my radar. I could scarcely believe that this is how my career would ultimately end, being sent home, weeping, in the back seat of a taxi, the last trip home I'd ever take from work.

The ability to return to work after a serious cardiac event can hinge on several factors. Many heart patients I know recuperate uneventfully at home for a few weeks and are able to return happily back to work with only limited restrictions, almost as if nothing's happened. Some attempt a return-to-work trial as I did, but find it impossible to keep up with the physical or mental demands required of the job. Depending on the severity of the heart condition, damage to heart muscle or valves, and ongoing cardiac issues, this may mean permanent retirement, a change to part-time employment, applying for a disability pension, or a significant career change to a much different occupation. If you're un-sure, talk to your physician about any limitations your own diagnosis may have on your ability to return to work.

The decision to apply for a disability pension is often not really a decision at all. It's an end-of-the-road last resort when you've run out of all other options, short of depleting your life savings. When I was at Mayo Clinic after my heart attack in 2008, I met American heart patients who had lost their jobs, their homes, or their family businesses because of catastrophic medical bills they were still trying to pay off from their last hospitalization. This is a truly desperate way to live, never mind trying to recuperate from a health crisis at the same time. If you lose your job, you lose your ability to pay those medical bills and support your family.

Depending on where you live, there are generally two basic types of standard disability program definitions:

♥ assessed as unable to work at your current employment
♥ assessed as unable to work at any form of employment

My assessment was for the latter. The day that I was finally forced to apply for my own disability pension was one of the bleakest and most humiliating points in my life. I had to ask a friend to help me fill out the thick pile of paperwork because I was simply unable to focus on what the words on the pages meant. The first page we pulled out of the large brown envelope was a blank application to appeal a denial of disability benefits. Putting this page on the top meant only one thing to me: you can go through this application process, honey, but you'll need this appeal letter when we turn you down.

I now believe that working versus not working is a matter of perceived control. For example, had I decided years before my heart attack that I wanted to retire in my fifties, stay at home, launch a blog, and write a book, leaving the public relations career I loved might have seemed like a momentous milestone celebrated with a farewell party and congratulatory speeches—instead of like the failure to appropriately recuperate that it seemed at the time.

Ironically, the end result would have been exactly the same. But the decision to retire early was made for me, without me, while I wept in hot, feeble protest. This lack of choice meant that the outcome seemed so much harder to accept.

Some heart disease survivors discover that the cardiac event itself has been so life-changing that it prompts a brand-new look at all personal goals and dreams, far beyond work. A survivor of multiple heart attacks, for example, told me that after her last heart trauma, she made some wholesale changes in her life. She decided to quit her stressful job and divorced the "layabout slug" she was married to (her words, not mine), and is now working part-time leading architectural walking tours of her historic neighborhood and volunteering for her local branch of the American Heart Association.

A Heart Patient's Bucket List

Speaking of decisions, let's revisit the popular concept of the Bucket List—that Hollywood invention of wonderful things we really must do before we finally kick the bucket. Since surviving my heart attack, I've been asked on occasion by friends and family (and even people who barely know me) about my own Bucket List. Because I have survived what many do not, they wonder if:

♥ I now have a greater determination to live every moment to the fullest?

♥ I plan to experience all those adventures I may have put off until now?

♥ I have created a list of exciting life-affirming goals to achieve before I head off to that great Coronary Care Unit in the sky?

The answer is an unqualified "No!" In fact, I sincerely doubt that I'd actually be any happier than I am right at this moment if only I could go bungee jumping / skydiving / bull riding / Everest climbing. My personal belief has long been that I always have enough time, enough money, and enough energy to do what I really, really want to do. When I look back on my life, that belief has been confirmed over and over again. So if I haven't done it by now, I'm thinking that, based on results, it simply wasn't that important to me after all. If it had been, the truth is that I would have already found some way, somehow, to get it done.

My great cardiac adventure did have a profound impact on my life in so many ways, but none of that impact resulted in creating a Bucket List. Instead, it merely reinforced what I'd long known already: that I must spend the very precious few hours I have left here on Earth (whether that's a big or a small number) doing far more of what I love doing, and far less of what I don't. Generally speaking, this means that how we spend our days is in fact how we spend our lives. Today, right at this moment—not someday, one day, maybe, down the road, or just in time before we kick that bucket.

But perhaps the most important reason I don't need a Bucket List: I hate making To Do lists and don't want to add anything more onto any of them.

One morning, for example, a few months after my heart attack, I had only two tasks on that day's entire To Do list:

1. a doctor's appointment
2. a stop at the farmer's market on the way home

But that latter task actually took me three exhausting days. As a heart patient living with ongoing symptoms, I apparently have enough energy to shop for several canvas bags of produce, clean out the fridge to make room for all this new stuff, and prep / pack away all the incoming fruit and veggies—just not all on the same day.

A Bucket List seems like merely a fancy-schmancy To Do list with major deadline pressure, created by people who aren't already doing what they love doing in life. And each item on this list must really deserve to be there. Not just an ordinary plan that makes you happy: "I think I'd like to go to the bead shop and make a couple of bracelets this weekend." Oh, no . . .

It seems that all itemized Bucket List goals must include Big Things like a fabulous vacation. But vacation travel is simply no longer on any of my To Do lists. After far too many years spent traveling on business during my corporate PR career, I've already exceeded my lifetime quota of time wasted on delayed flights and car rentals, fretting over lost luggage, drinking bad coffee, eating weird food, trying in vain to get a good night's sleep in too many strange beds, using scary toilets, standing in endlessly long lines, making cheery small talk with strangers I'll never see again, and recuperating from jet lag. And don't even get me started on flights filled with loud drunks, ever-shrinking leg room, and that kid who keeps kicking the back of your seat.

Whenever I contemplate all those vacation scenarios, especially as a person living with a chronic illness, I feel the need for a wee lie-down until the urge to leave town passes. Whenever I'm invited to speak at a faraway conference (i.e., one that requires more than a ferry ride to Vancouver), I ask myself how willing I am to sacrifice my carefully balanced daily functional capacity for a too-brief time onstage. And more importantly, I wonder how many board-certified cardiologists will be in my audience, just in case.

If I never again see the inside of another airport, that will be just dandy with me. Besides, I live in Lotus Land here on the magnificent West Coast of Canada, arguably the most gorgeous spot on earth. People from around the world save up their money all year long just to be able to vacation here. Why would I ever want to leave? And remember, as Buddhist wisdom reminds us, wherever you go, there you are.

If you decide to create your own shiny new Bucket List because you've recently survived a catastrophic wake-up call, it's important to keep your expectations in check. Successfully ticking off the items on your list may not fill you with the supremely satisfying exhilaration you believe it will. Just imagine how horrible you'd feel if you actually did accomplish one of your ultimate Bucket List goals—let's say, completing a triathlon—and it turned out to be an even uglier experience than a triathlon normally is.

Bucket lists by definition represent more of something we don't already have at the moment, but somehow believe that if only we could have it / buy it / do it / eat it / see it / experience it, we would really, finally, truly be happy. That seductive word *more* traps us in our own sense of the perpetual dissatisfaction we may feel for not having quite enough yet.

This is also an embarrassingly unique First-World problem, dear readers. I'm guessing that very few refugees fleeing war-torn combat zones are checking their Bucket Lists today.

As a heart patient who is simply trying to navigate step by step through this new normal of living with a chronic illness diagnosis, it seems that our only actual sure-fire road to happiness might well be accompanied by finding joy in the pure and basic pleasures of day-to-day life, and by keeping our expectations low.

And by not making Bucket Lists.

Are You Too Hard on Yourself?

Coming to grips with this new normal after a major health crisis sometimes includes lots of self-blame and regret. Being hard on ourselves can be especially common after a cardiac event or a medical diagnosis that might be viewed as self-inflicted:

I should have quit smoking earlier.
Maybe if I'd done a better job controlling my blood pressure.
Why didn't I listen to my doctor's advice?
If only I'd kept those New Year's resolutions to exercise more!

When I was a little girl in the 1950s, my parents were stingy with praise and magnanimous with criticism. To be otherwise could result in a child developing an inflated ego, which, as all parents knew back then, would be the worst possible thing that could ever happen to any kid. "She really thinks she's a somebody!" was a phrase delivered with withering contempt by my mother in describing any person whose sense of self-esteem seemed even remotely healthy.

Nobody, according to my parents, likes a kid with a swelled head. The only way to prevent that catastrophe was to be tough on your children, and in turn teach them to be equally tough on themselves. You could thus help them avoid growing up to be spoiled adults who went around acting like they were a somebody.

But another approach (not ever approved by my mother) is self-compassion, a central construct in Buddhist psychology. It means being warm and understanding toward ourselves when we're suffering, rather than ignoring our pain or beating ourselves up with self-criticism. Dr. Kristin Neff teaches educational psychology at the University of

Texas at Austin and is the author of the book *Self-Compassion*. She explains that children who grow up like I did can end up experiencing very little self-compassion when life's difficulties strike in adulthood.

> Instead of mercilessly judging and criticizing yourself for various inadequacies or shortcomings, self-compassion means you are kind and understanding when confronted with personal failings— after all, who ever said you were supposed to be perfect? You may try to change in ways that allow you to be more healthy and happy, but this is done because you care about yourself, not because you're unacceptable as you are.[18]

She suggests that, instead of ignoring our pain with stiff-upper-lip determination, we should stop and think, "This is really difficult for me right now. How can I comfort and care for myself in this moment?"[19]

Because having a heart attack is such a profoundly life-altering event for most survivors, we now get many opportunities to practice self-compassion daily—although in my case, I have to tell you that my own experience with this foreign concept was a disaster at the beginning. During the weeks and months post-op, I mostly just felt despair and anxiety over my inexplicable failure to bounce right back. "What's wrong with you?" I would wail silently to that exhausted stranger's face in the mirror.

I wish that I'd known then about the value of self-compassion when facing challenges like a chronic illness diagnosis. But it's never too late to re-learn how to be kinder to ourselves. We might, however, have to consciously unlearn lifelong habits while developing the new habit of self-compassion, as Dr. Neff suggests: "Self-compassion also requires taking a balanced approach to our negative emotions so that feelings are neither suppressed nor exaggerated."[20]

So go ahead. Be a somebody, because you are.

10 ♡ Making Peace with an Errant Organ

Here's my theory: few health crises in life are as traumatic as surviving a cardiac event. I developed this theory while I was busy having my own heart attack in the spring of 2008.

Experiencing a heart attack feels so unimaginably surreal that I, like many heart patients, try extremely hard to deny those first symptoms when they strike out of the blue. After being misdiagnosed with acid reflux by a confident (yet mistaken) ER physician, I kept trying to ignore those symptoms for two terrible weeks until they were no longer bearable. I forced myself back to the ER for help, this time for an accurate diagnosis.

I now know that almost two-thirds of women who die during a heart attack have never experienced any previous cardiac symptoms.[1] A report published in the World Heart Federation's journal *Global Heart* suggests that, compared to our male counterparts, women are twice as likely to die within one year, even if we do survive the initial heart attack.[2]

If—and sadly, each of these is still a great big fat if—we survive the actual cardiac event, and if we are near a hospital that's able to provide an experienced team of cardiologists / cardiothoracic surgeons / cardiac nurses / technologists, and if we are correctly diagnosed, and if we receive timely and appropriate treatment, and if the resulting damage to our oxygen-deprived heart muscle is not too severe, we finally get to go home.

Although I don't know this at the time I'm discharged from the hospital, I am soon to discover that the emotional fallout of a traumatic health crisis such as a heart attack often waits to strike until much later.

Post–Heart Attack Stun

I did survive that heart attack—but my initial relief at being alive was quickly replaced by what Jodi Jackson likes to call Post–Heart Attack Stun. Jodi was only 42 years old when she had the same type of cardiac event that I experienced, that oddly named widow maker heart attack. In her guest post for Jen Thorson's *My Life in Red* blog, Jodi described Post–Heart Attack Stun as the period following a cardiac crisis in which "everything seems so surreal that you can't really absorb what has just happened."[3]

Jodi started showing the first signs of Stun in 2011 at her home near Kansas City. "That day, I started feeling bad on the way home from work. By the time I got home, I knew I was really sick. Trying to deny it, I changed clothes and took the dog out."[4]

It turns out that changing out of your work clothes and taking the dog for a walk is not an uncommon reaction in women experiencing a heart attack. So is driving the kids to soccer, finishing that report, cooking Christmas dinner, or flying to Ottawa, apparently. In Jodi's case, she knew by the time she got back into the house with the dog that she did need to call an ambulance because of the unusual heaviness in her chest and the searing pain in her lower jaw. She put the dog in its crate, and called 911. She was told to chew an aspirin and swallow it while she waited for the ambulance. That's when the Stun hit again: "The ambulance arrived, and my husband, who was out of town, called at the same time. I told him I couldn't talk because the paramedics were there, and I hung up the phone."

At the hospital, Jodi learned she was having a massive heart attack. Three coronary stents were implanted. Like me, she could scarcely believe her symptoms had been heart related. As she explained, "It's hard to absorb any of it because although I knew I'd had a heart attack, I didn't feel like it. The symptoms I had experienced were nothing like what I thought a heart attack would be because I never lost consciousness."

I actually laughed out loud at Jodi's description of what happened to her later that evening, when, alone in her hospital room, she decided to phone her longtime friend, Deb.

Deb: "Hey, what are you up to?"

Jodi: "I just had a heart attack."

Deb: "Over what?"

Jodi: "Seriously, I just had a heart attack. I just got out of the cath lab!"

Deb: (Stunned silence)

I knew instantly what Jodi meant by Post–Heart Attack Stun. During my second trip to the ER, my own brain had shut down the minute I heard the cardiologist saying, "You have significant heart disease."

Even while recuperating from treatment in the hospital, I seemed to be living in a not unpleasant type of La La Land. I knew I'd been moved to the coronary care unit (CCU, cardiology's intensive care ward), I knew that a major artery in my heart had been blocked, and I'd heard the CCU nurses using the term STEMI, which I knew meant heart attack. But I still felt confused enough to keep asking the nurses what they had meant, just in case the diagnosis might have been downgraded since my admission.

Physicians and nurses would do well to remember this state of Post–Heart Attack Stun while they're breaking bad news or explaining details of a significant cardiac event to their patients—even to those of us who are politely nodding as if we're truly able to comprehend them.

Years later, I was transported back to those surreal early moments in the CCU while watching the final few scenes of the Tom Hanks movie *Captain Phillips*. It's based on the harrowing true story of an American cargo ship hijacked by Somali pirates in 2009. In the film's final minutes, Captain Phillips, finally rescued from his horrific ordeal, is taken to a military ship's infirmary to get checked. He's so overwhelmed by what he's just survived that he can barely make out what the medic is saying.[5]

Although essentially unhurt physically, Phillips appears unable to understand or respond to the routine questions she's asking him. But suddenly, the enormity of what's happened hits home. Although Hanks as Captain Phillips has remained a paragon of composure throughout the hijacking crisis, he now begins to cry. He can't stop crying. And there I was, crying right along with him in that darkened theater, big snotty crying sobs, recalling my own inability to understand the unintelligible noises coming at me while hospitalized years earlier.

Health care providers must pay close attention to the real-life emotional, mental, and psychological trauma embodied in the whole person they are treating, trauma that can morph all communication into a sort of muffled bad dream while patients struggle to comprehend the incomprehensible.

Here's what would have helped both me and Captain Phillips. When confronting a shocked and stunned patient in the throes of a crisis, doctors and nurses could take a deep breath before offering a long explanation or a list of questions. Speak clearly, slowly, and plainly. Don't use medical jargon that most patients wouldn't understand even if they weren't in crisis.

Meanwhile, here are some sound suggestions from Mayo Clinic to help patients get past this surreal post-diagnosis shock once we get home:

♥ Honestly examine what you fear.
♥ Think about the potential negative consequences of not taking action.
♥ Allow yourself to express your fears and emotions.
♥ Try to identify irrational beliefs about your situation.
♥ Journal about your experience in writing.
♥ Open up to a trusted friend or loved one.
♥ Participate in a support group with other patients.
♥ Learn as much as you can about your new diagnosis.[6]

The Loss of Self

Eventually, reality had a nasty way of intruding into my dogged refusal to come to grips with what had just happened to me, piercing even my most protective Post–Heart Attack Stun response. Leaving the hospital gave way to the shock of being back at home, almost as if none of that drama had actually happened. But heart disease immediately and profoundly began to affect my quality of life. My well-being, career,

A Letter to My Pre–Heart Attack Self

I've learned a thing or two since 2008 about living with a chronic and progressive illness. I wish it hadn't taken a heart attack to learn them. I think I might have been a nicer, smarter, or kinder person had I known these things back then. So in no particular order, here's a list of my best advice to that long-ago me:

Dear Carolyn,

Don't waste time worrying about answers to every question. (Sometimes, we simply don't know the answers to all questions—like "Why me? Why did this happen?" Relentless navel-gazing can end up being crazy-making—and it's boring to others.)

Don't be smug. (Just because you've been a healthy distance runner for almost two decades, don't believe that this somehow provides a magical cardioprotective guarantee against having a heart attack one day.)

Don't be so damned judgmental. (You know absolutely nothing about the life of that chubby guy eating ice cream, or that mother yelling at her kids in the mall, or that heart patient who starts smoking again until you have walked a mile in their hospital booties.)

Don't take your family and friends for granted. (You have no idea how important those you love really are until you need them someday during a real crisis.) But conversely . . .

Don't squander the precious and limited hours you have left on this Earth with people who suck the life right out of you. (You may have always believed that you had little choice in the need to spend time with some of these folks, but trust me, you'll be far healthier if you try to keep interactions with them to a bare minimum.)

Don't live to work. (Stop bragging about how crazy-busy you are at work. Stop doing nutty workaholic things like going into the office every Sunday for the last year before your heart attack in order to stay on top of all those important projects—

trust me, nobody on their deathbed will ever say, "Wish I'd spent more time at the office.")

Don't interject unsolicited opinions—until somebody absolutely begs you, but even then practice more listening instead. (Your opinion is just that, an opinion—not the Capital T Truth—so resist the urge to share.) Please note: as my family and friends can attest, I'm still working hard on this one . . .

Don't be reluctant to ask for (and then accept) help from others who offer. (Most people wouldn't offer if they didn't really want to help you—and you know how good you feel when you can do something kind for others in need. Allow others the same pleasure.)

Don't ever believe that bad things don't happen to good people. (There is no Fair Fairy in life, so stop acting as if those who get sick are somehow not like you because, unlike them, you are smart enough, strong enough, fit enough, committed enough, or educated enough to outrun hurt and pain and illness. You can't. Try being nicer to those who are finding that out for themselves.)

Don't try for Best Patient award. (There is none—and the choices you make won't be the same as those made by others with the same diagnosis anyway, and that's okay. You are not them. Being sick doesn't make you more noble or more special— it just makes you feel really bad some days and not so bad on other days. It is what it is.)

Don't neglect the beauty of unremarkable routine. (Take a longer, more scenic walk home from work. Always keep fresh flowers on your desk. Listen to Barber's Adagio for Strings every day.)

Best of luck to you, Carolyn,

Love,

Your future self

finances, personal relationships, and especially my sense of self were soon to be turned upside down and inside out.

When California sociologist Dr. Kathy Charmaz studied people living with chronic illness, she identified something that's often overlooked by health care providers. In her research published in the journal *Sociology of Health and Illness*, Dr. Charmaz warned that a narrow medicalized view of suffering (defined only as physical symptoms) can minimize the broader significance of suffering in those of us diagnosed with a chronic and progressive illness such as heart disease:

> A fundamental form of that suffering is the loss of self in chronically ill persons who observe their former self images crumbling away without the simultaneous development of equally valued new ones. The experiences and meanings upon which these ill persons had built former positive self images are no longer available to them.[7]

I was very moved when I read about this loss of self. Dr. Charmaz captured precisely what I'd been feeling, too. The self I had known—at home, at work, socially, professionally—indeed had seemed to be crumbling away as debilitating cardiac symptoms continued, and then worsened. My doctors continued to search for ways to address my chest pain, shortness of breath, and crushing fatigue, but nothing seemed to work. My life had become so different from my pre–heart attack days that the self I lived with now was almost unrecognizable to me.

This shift in reality isn't applicable only to heart patients. Dr. Charmaz's research included those living with at least one of a range of chronic diagnoses, including cardiovascular disease, diabetes, cancer, multiple sclerosis, and lupus. Hers is one of the most comprehensive overviews of the psychosocial toll accompanying chronic illness that I've found.

She suggested that this loss of self can actually start early—sometimes even before an official diagnosis is made—and can continue to grow from there as the illness progresses. For example:

♥ *Pre-diagnosis:* The first impact on my sense of self struck as the ER physician misdiagnosed me when I sought help for my earliest cardiac symptoms. I left the hospital that morning feeling embarrassed because I'd just made a big fuss over nothing, and stupid because I clearly wasn't capable of figuring out the difference between a heart attack and plain old indigestion. Dr. Charmaz warns that physicians sometimes dismiss undiagnosed people "as neurotics whose symptoms are either nonexistent or psychosomatic in origin, leaving the patients feeling unsupported or guilty for having brought their discomfort upon themselves."[8]

♥ *Beginning of illness:* Family and friends are often extremely attentive when the shocking news of a health crisis first breaks, but their involvement understandably fades as they return to their own busy lives. This is to be expected, says Dr. Charmaz: "As time goes by, such attention generally tends to dwindle."[9]

♥ *Concern about burdening others:* I could see firsthand how alarmed my family and friends were by what had just happened to me, so I tried to smile my bravest happy smile around them so they could stop worrying. Dr. Charmaz observed comparable reactions in her study, including several married women who expressed "a fear of greater impairment since their husbands did not like sick people."[10]

♥ *Limitation of life:* It took me a surprisingly long time to learn how to carefully restrict my usual daily activities in order to preserve my ability to function. But as Dr. Charmaz explains, "When people are forced into limiting normal activities to protect their health, they may do so at great costs to one's self-image. Most importantly, living a restricted life can foster an all-consuming retreat into illness."[11]

♥ *Unpredictability:* I was thunderstruck by how hard it was to predict when I might have a good day or a bad day, or even intermittent bad spells during any given day. I would make—but then need to cancel on short notice—countless plans due to symptom flares. According to Dr. Charmaz, "Due to their unpredictable conditions, patients can suffer disruptions of their lives and selves that go far beyond physical discomfort. Such disruptions may include the necessity of quitting work, limiting social engagements, or avoiding activity."[12]

♥ *Work:* Some heart patients feel well enough to bounce right back to the office relatively quickly, while others, like me, are no longer able to return to work. Coping with either decision can affect our sense of self, says Dr. Charmaz. "When fortunate enough to work, persons living with chronic illness frequently feel they have to restrict all other activities in order to manage the demands of their jobs. But when forced to leave work, they may be reduced to leaving their prior social worlds entirely."[13]

♥ *All-consuming focus:* It was almost impossible for me to keep trying to act as though everything was fine when it was so clearly untrue. It's hard to focus on much else when living with distressing symptoms. "Serious illness can flood identity," Dr. Charmaz adds. "Illness becomes the focus of life as treatment regimens, living with constant discomfort, medical appointments, and the problems of mundane activities structure and fill the day."[14]

Dr. Charmaz believes that the world seems set up for the healthy and able—a reality that those living with a chronic illness usually don't even question. She also believes that this reality helps to explain why the people she studies so often judge themselves by yardsticks more appropriately applied to the healthy and able. I believe that, too. As we see happening within the concept of healthy privilege, it's the healthy, able people out there who own the yardsticks in the first place.

What's in store for patients who fear that their sense of self is truly slipping away?

For me, I sensed a gradual but steady improvement after I finally found a good therapist to talk about what was happening to me. In this person, I found a willing and compassionate ear, but also a no-nonsense source of grounded perspective on my conflicting emotions. I know that Dr. Barbara Keddy (who, in chapter 7, warned us not to obsess over our diagnosis by talking about it all the time with family and friends) would probably approve of the way we almost never talked about heart disease during therapy appointments, preferring to focus on how I was planning to address, for example, my deep reluctance to say "No" to people, and how to accommodate and rearrange the new normal that had become my life. As it turned out, these were likely the issues I most needed to focus on.

Speaking of saying "No," the truth is that until recently, I've spent much of my adult life saying "Yes!" to things, even when I didn't really want to. For example, I used to let other people dictate my social calendar. When they asked, "Are you free on Friday evening?," I'd almost always agree to their plans for me if my calendar happened to be blank. Before I knew what had hit me, on Friday evening I'd often be on my way to an event I didn't really want to attend, with people I didn't really want to be with, while at the same time missing out on activities or people I preferred, and wondering, "What am I doing here?"

But now, living with ongoing cardiac symptoms, I knew that I somehow had to clearly redefine how I would choose to spend those precious few hours of feeling well I might have each day. I could no longer allow others to decide how I invested my time. My therapist and I came up with this solution: in my purse calendar, the week-at-a-glance kind, I write the word "NO!" on the top of each page. When somebody asks, "Are you free on Friday?," I now reply, "Let me check my calendar." And when I do, there in big bold caps, I'll find the word "NO!" This doesn't mean I decline every invitation, but it's a useful reminder simply to pause and think carefully about whether or not this particular use of my time is what will support my health right now. If it doesn't, I say, "I just checked my calendar and—no! I'm not free." No explanation, no apology, no discussion required.

Sometimes, living with a chronic and progressive illness means giving up the control we've had until now over almost every basic daily decision. I believe that regaining control of decision making, even small decisions, might help to stem that loss of self, the "crumbling away" of our former self-image, as Dr. Charmaz calls it.[15]

Just remember that "No!" is a complete sentence.

Ready for Talk Therapy?

If you are a heart patient who's thinking about making an appointment for talk therapy, it's important to seek out a professional who is experienced in working specifically with chronically ill patients. If your heart hospital has cardiac social workers or cardiac psychologists on staff to help you, even better.

We know that this kind of specialized therapy is effective in other areas of medicine as well. When I worked in hospice palliative care, for example, we had a large staff of skilled bereavement counselors who are familiar with end-of-life issues and are trained in providing care for patients until death, and then for their surviving family members long afterward. These people have a depth of understanding of, and specialize in, grief issues.

My friends who have undergone cancer treatment tell me that they, too, found immense relief in being able to talk to the staff psychologists working at the cancer hospital. These people are already familiar with experiences and emotions unique to their clients, from cancer diagnosis through treatment and beyond to what they call survivorship (the part of your life after treatment ends). Their depth of understanding is specialized for cancer issues.

In both examples, clients don't have to start from zero to bring their counselors up to speed, because a type of condition-specific shorthand already exists that can help them get right to the meat of each conversation.

By comparison, the first counselor I saw briefly (before finding the very helpful one I later stayed with for many months) was the contract psychologist whose services were provided free of charge for a limited number of visits as part of our extended health employee benefits package at work. But she seemed to know nothing whatsoever about what it's like to be diagnosed with heart disease or anything else. I felt as though I was spending an exasperatingly long time just explaining to her the basics of cardiology, instead of getting around to the reason I really wanted to consult a psychologist in the first place. The last straw was when, during our third appointment, she cheerfully said to me these exact words: "I know! Why don't you sign up to take an interesting course at the university?"

I almost fell off the brown plaid chair I was sitting on. Take an interesting university course? Hadn't she heard a word I'd said for three weeks? I was barely able to brush my teeth and get myself across town for these appointments. I wasn't depressed because I needed a fun class in mid-century modern architecture. I was depressed because I'd just had a frickety-fracking heart attack!

That visit marked the end of our therapeutic relationship, but luckily, that meant a space opened for the next one, a far more appropriate match who also had decades of experience in chronic illness. Sometimes you need to shop around before finding a good fit for such an important undertaking. The second therapist reminded me, for example, that although much had changed in my life because of heart disease, all of my instincts were still intact (albeit temporarily buried under denial and incapacitated by fear). But over time, she helped me to believe that I was capable of digging them up.

This belief was the beginning of finding that lost self.

The Enemy Within

One of my *Heart Sisters* blog readers—a double-whammy winner in the Sweepstakes of Truly Awful Diagnoses (first breast cancer and then, five years later, heart disease)—wrote to me about how her heart attack had differed significantly from her cancer experience. "With cancer, the enemy was something foreign that had somehow invaded my body. A tumor should not be there, and all medical effort is intensely focused on getting rid of this evil intruder. But with heart disease, the threat comes from my own heart, from part of me. I can't get rid of that!"[16]

Those living with other chronic illnesses have lobbed similar accusations against their own errant bowels, pancreas, lungs, joints, and other assorted body parts that simply do not work like the owner's manual promised. My reader's observation echoed this surprisingly common reaction among many heart attack survivors: the belief that our hearts have somehow betrayed us.

That word *betray* is also how the late physician, author, and Yale professor Dr. Sherwin Nuland once described a heart attack during a presentation to a Seattle audience: "So commonly do coronary arteries betray the heart whose muscle they are meant to sustain, that their treachery is the cause of at least half of North American deaths. Each time a person recovers from a heart attack of any size, he or she has lost a little more muscle to the increasing area of scar tissue."[17]

Now there's a cheerful sentiment for you. The trust we have had that this heart will continue to beat regularly and pump blood like it's supposed to do, something that we've taken for granted all our lives, has suddenly evaporated. Unlike that breast cancer patient who feared the external danger that had invaded her body, heart patients fear the danger that lives within.

And after my own heart's betrayal, each little cramp, ache, or twinge in my chest felt every bit as alarming as the first symptoms that forced me to seek emergency care.

Anger Raises Its Ugly Head

I returned home as a freshly diagnosed heart patient keen to return to my normal routine, but rapidly realized that any sense of normal seemed to have vanished. Anger is often one of the many emotional reactions to this kind of realization, often the first to break through any last vestiges of what Jodi Jackson calls our Post–Heart Attack Stun. But just wait until another penny drops: the knowledge that one of the most significant risk factors for having a heart attack is having already had one.

Sometimes heart disease survivors can feel upset or angry at themselves, especially if they, or somebody they care about, suspects that their own lifestyle choices might be at least partly responsible for what's just happened, that this diagnosis was somehow self-inflicted.

Anger is so common following a cardiac event, in fact, that the American Heart Association (AHA) now warns that erupting feelings of post-diagnosis anger can threaten both our current recovery as well as our risk of having another cardiac event. That's why it's important to understand these feelings, recognize problems before they get too big, and seek professional help when needed. As the AHA explains: "Many heart patients feel angry and upset about what's happened to them. But anger can cause your blood pressure and heart rate to rise, and make your heart work harder. Sometimes anger also causes angina (chest pain) because blood vessels narrow, reducing blood flow and oxygen to the heart muscle."[18]

Depending on personal circumstances, the anger of heart patients is directed not just at themselves, but at one or more distinct targets, including:

♥ at an unruly organ that has suddenly let us down (All those years, I believed that my heart was perfectly healthy!)
♥ at the unfairness of life (Why me? I've been doing everything right!)
♥ at our loved ones (Stop treating me like an invalid!)
♥ at a health care system that has failed us (How could that doctor have misdiagnosed me and sent me home from the ER despite those textbook symptoms?)
♥ at the new routine that requires us to do what we don't want to do (All these pills? Another doctor's appointment? And now cardiac rehab classes?)

Sometimes being angry with others—or at yourself—is a way of covering up underlying fear and anxiety, something that many of us have lots of during recovery. And by the way, anger toward others can easily expand to include people we don't even know.

I went through a strange period like this in the early days after my dad, a non-smoker, died at age 62 of metastatic lung cancer. For a time after his death, I noticed that I was becoming really annoyed at old people. All old people. Any old people. I'd watch them with barely concealed outrage while they shuffled slowly across the street. How could these useless old people still be alive when my own fit and vibrant father was dead?

Jenni Grover Prokopy, the author of *ChronicBabe 101: How to Craft an Incredible Life beyond Illness* and founder of the blog *Chronic Babe*, writes frequently about patients' emotions, including anger, which she believes are completely normal among those living with a serious health condition. I love her take on anger:

Diagnosis of a chronic illness is one of the most stressful life events we can imagine. Even 20 years since my own diagnosis, I can still get angry. But my solution is coming back to the concept of acceptance, recognizing that illness is part of my life and isn't going anywhere.

If we fight our illness when we're angry at ourselves and at our body for being sick, we're fighting facts, we're fighting with ourselves, fighting things we don't have control over. Getting angry at our illness causes self-harm. And don't we already have enough pain and suffering without causing ourselves more anger at our situation?[19]

Jenni adds that she also relies on a helpful and supportive team described as "friends, family, my manicurist, my mailman, and anybody who will hear me out and not let me host an enormous pity party."

Speaking of those pity parties, a good place to avoid their seductive pull is in the kind of pull-up-your-socks advice that heart attack survivor Jen Thorson dishes out on her blog, *My Life in Red:*

I have little patience with willful ignorance of cardiac risk factors (just as I do for "being embarrassed" as the reason someone doesn't seek care). I've done this survivor/writer/speaker thing long enough and heard enough stories to just be over that. I get it, I do, but ladies, we need to get beyond it. We need to take control of our health and care. No one else is going to do it for us.[20]

If it starts to feel as though anger is affecting your relationships with others and/or your health, please consider seeking professional help. Short-term anger can easily morph into a toxic long-term resentful worldview. This is not only damaging to physical health, but it can mean that the only people who will want to be around you are other angry people. Don't let that happen to you.

Yes, You Will Be Happy Again

Some people, particularly those who have recently been diagnosed with heart disease, might argue that of course they can't feel happy right now. How can they possibly be happy in the middle of such a serious health crisis? Dr. Sonja Lyubomirsky, an internationally known researcher, author, and professor of psychology at the University of California Riverside, has a unique perspective on this possibility. (By the way, her last name, in a neat twist of karmic perfection if you're a person who studies happiness, comes from the Russian words for love and peace.)

Dr. Lyubomirsky knows a lot about happiness, but teaches two key lessons that seem especially relevant to heart patients. In a 2014 lecture at California's Pepperdine University, she explained that we actually have a genetic predisposition to be happy or not, and also that our level of happiness can be changed by how we behave and how we think about what's happening to us.[21]

Rather than life events shaping our outlook, her research suggests that it's more likely the other way around: our outlook actually shapes how we respond to life events. She warns, however, that this can take work. It may be tough for the freshly diagnosed to believe this in the early days or weeks of surviving a health crisis, but Dr. Lyubomirsky assures us:

> Life's turning points do not have to become major crises after all. In fact, our research has found that life events do not have much of an impact on optimism or happiness. And as crazy as this might seem, I recognize one true thing: the older we get (except maybe for extreme old age), the better the chances of being able to handle any given catastrophe, entirely due to all those years of experience in successfully handling all kinds of difficult problems, big and small.[22]

Her words rang true for me. In my experience with heart disease, I learned to cope with crisis by coping. I learned to adapt to crisis by adapting. I learned to roll with the punches because, like so many of us, I've practiced rolling with so many figurative punches during my life. It's not because I needed the crisis to become a better person, not because the diagnosis itself was some kind of a gift, and certainly not because I needed to add meaning to a meaningless existence, but because I now believe that all human beings have a remarkable ability to get used to almost anything in life (both positive and negative).

Dr. Lyubomirsky's research also suggests that what happens to you in life actually doesn't seem to matter as much as you might expect. We sometime hear things such as, "I'm not very happy now, but I will be happy as soon as I _____" (fill in the blank: get married, get divorced, get that job, quit this job, buy this, sell that, recuperate from this cardiac event, etc.). But she reminds us that when we actually get what we think will make us happy, we will quickly adapt to that new thing, and then we'll start taking it for granted. We actually feel far less happy about getting it than we'd hoped.

Her research also suggests that, although most people dread going through a really bad experience (getting fired from your job or the death of a spouse, for example), about four to five years after the bad experience happens, measurable happiness indicators actually show that people are often as happy as they were before the experience, and often even happier.

Dr. Lyubomirsky adds that happy people also tend to have certain traits in common compared to generally unhappy people—and it's not because happy people don't have their fair share of dreadful problems. They're more likely to exercise regularly, to practice acts of kindness, to invest in relationships, to practice their religion, to be forgiving, to nurture optimistic thinking, to meditate, and to cope well with adversity. (And maybe they're coping well with adversity because of all that other stuff they're doing first.)

Social psychologist Dr. Martin Seligman suggests that gratitude, for some people, might be a loaded word when you're trying to cope with adversity. So instead of asking what his severely depressed clients and research subjects are grateful for (they'll answer "Nothing!"), he asks them to simply write down three good things that have happened that day. As he once told a *Time* magazine interviewer, "If you have people every night write down three things that went well that day and why, six months later these people will report more happiness and less depression."[23]

Dr. Seligman also talked about a common-sense concept called emotional contagion. The more time you spend with unhappy, pessimistic people, he says, the more you'll feel the same way yourself. He adds that the opposite has been shown to be true, too. Substitute happy, optimistic companions, and you'll feel happier just being around them. This also seems like a sound argument not only for avoiding isolation, but more importantly, for thinking carefully about how you choose your companions.

Thanking My Brave Little Heart

Before you think we're getting too far ahead of ourselves in a rush toward all this bubbly happiness, let's remember that no matter how many times new heart patients are reassured that our negative, weepy, angry, or fearful reactions are normal, trust me when I tell you that anxiety about dying represents a relentlessly exhausting way to live—and all because the body's most important organ has stopped doing what we trust it to do.

That exhaustion is what ultimately led me to a Eureka! moment of patienthood, inspired by a lovely person named Heather Fox. Heather is a wise, caring friend and former hospice colleague who visited me at home in those early weeks post–heart attack. I was pretty much of a mess at the time, unsuccessfully trying to make sense of debilitating symptoms that had not yet been correctly diagnosed as coronary microvascular disease, and struggling emotionally over what was happening to my life. I had very few words of appreciation for a body part that had let me down in such spectacular fashion, until one day when Heather, an experienced grief counselor, brought me a little gift.

The gift was one of those guided imagery tapes meant for recent heart attack survivors. For several calming minutes of softly tinkling music in the background, the voice on the tape invited me to quietly visualize oxygenated blood cells coursing happily through my newly revascularized coronary arteries. Instead of letting me continue to blame my heart for messing up its only job, Heather's challenge was to change how I fundamentally thought about and talked to my own heart. Instead of resenting my heart for letting me down, I was now asked to say:

"I thank my brave little heart for helping me survive what so many do not."

That single message has stuck with me every day since then (well, almost every day . . . on some days, let's face it, it's harder to remember that generous acknowledgement). But instead of blame, mistrust, anger, fear, and resentment—which had filled so much of my soul during those early "Why me?" days—I am getting much better at placing my hand over my chest several times a day now and offering this gentle whisper:

"Thank you."

My heart is not a perfect organ, and no amount of gratitude will ever change what's already happened to it, but given what it's been through on my behalf, my amazing and heroic little heart deserves my heartfelt gratitude.

Recommended Resources

Helpful Books for Heart Patients

Dr. James Beckerman, *Heart to Start* (Portland, OR: Providence Heart and Vascular Institute, 2015).

Toni Bernhard, *How to Be Sick: A Buddhist-Inspired Guide for the Chronically Ill and Their Caregivers* (Somerville: Wisdom Publications, 2010).

Toni Bernhard, *How to Live Well with Chronic Pain and Illness: A Mindful Guide* (Somerville, Wisdom Publications, 2015).

Bernard J. Gersh, *Mayo Clinic Heart Book, Second Edition* (New York: William Morrow, 2000).

Dr. Nieca Goldberg, *The Women's Healthy Heart Program: Lifesaving Strategies for Preventing and Healing Heart Disease* (New York: Ballantine Books, 2006).

Dr. Martha Gulati and Sherry Torkos, *Saving Women's Hearts* (Hoboken: Wiley, 2011).

Kathy Kastan, *From the Heart* (Cambridge, MA: Perseus, 2007).

Rhoda Levin, *Heartmates: A Survival Guide for the Cardiac Spouse* (New York: Pocket Books, 1987).

Dr. Wayne Sotile, *Heart Illness and Intimacy: How Caring Relationships Aid Recovery* (Baltimore: Johns Hopkins University Press, 1992).

Dr. Wayne Sotile, *Thriving with Heart Disease* (New York: Free Press, 2003).

Dr. Suzanne Steinbaum, *Dr. Suzanne Steinbaum's Heart Book: Every Woman's Guide to a Heart-Healthy Life* (New York: Avery, 2013).

Bonnie Stern, *HeartSmart: The Best of HeartSmart Cooking* (Toronto: Random House Canada, 2006).

Dr. Malissa Wood, *Smart at Heart: A Holistic 10-Step Approach to Preventing and Healing Heart Disease for Women* (Berkeley: Celestial Arts, 2011).

Helpful Websites for Heart Patients

Angioplasty.org: Founded by pioneers of interventional cardiology, this site has been a definitive source of information for physicians and a leading advocate for stent patients for 20 years, with over 12,000 posts on its influential Patient Forum. http://www.angioplasty.org.

Brugada Girl: Alicia Burns was a young mother when she was diagnosed with the rare heart rhythm disorder called Brugada Syndrome. Read her *Newly Diagnosed* posts if you're a newbie. https://brugadagirl.com/.

Chronic Babe: Jenni Grover Prokopy's articles, videos, and online community for younger women with chronic health issues who still want to lead an amazing life. http://www.chronicbabe.com/.

Dr. John M: Dr. John Mandrola is an electrophysiologist who treats heart rhythm problems. He writes, beautifully and clearly, about conditions such as atrial fibrillation, heart rhythm devices like pacemakers and ICDs, heart-healthy living, doctoring, and cycling. http://www.drjohnm.org/.

Go Red for Women: This awareness movement was launched by the American Heart Association to inform women about their risk of heart disease; best tool ever is the brilliant Elizabeth Banks 3-minute video called *"Just a Little Heart Attack."* https://www.goredforwomen.org/.

Heart and Stroke Foundation: A Canadian non-profit organization that offers info on healthy kids, great recipes, heart facts, and emerging cardiac research. www.heartandstroke.ca/.

Heart Sisters: My own blog, including over 700 articles on women's experience with heart disease, bridges the knowledge gap between patients and health care practitioners. It covers most of what's in this book and much more. www.myheartsisters.org/.

The Heart Truth: Sponsored by the National Heart, Lung and Blood Institute, this program aims to raise awareness about heart disease and its risk factors among women. http://www.nhlbi.nih.gov/health/educational/hearttruth/.

Mayo Clinic: My go-to favorite for basic heart disease info including symptoms, diagnostic tools, causes, risk factors, treatment, and prevention of many kinds of heart disease. http://www.mayoclinic.org/diseases-conditions/heart-disease/basics/definition/con-20034056.

Pumping Marvellous: A terrific UK site for people living with heart failure; includes patient self-management tools. Especially recommended for the newly diagnosed. http://pumpingmarvellous.org/.

StopAFib: For patients with atrial fibrillation; includes useful resources for both patients and caregivers. http://www.stopafib.org/.

WomenHeart: The National Coalition for Women with Heart Disease. Find a WomenHeart support group near you, an online support community, virtual support group meetings, and publications on many women's heart issues (including some in Spanish). http://www.womenheart.org/.

Notes

Preface

1. S. Koven, "Taking the Temperature of Sick Lit," interview with M. Enright, CBC Radio, *The Sunday Edition,* March 6, 2016, http://www.cbc.ca/1.3476189.

2. *Heart Sisters* (blog), http://www.myheartsisters.org.

3. Vancouver Coastal Health Research Institute, "Your Heart, Your Health," Vancouver, BC, May 24, 2015, http://www.vchri.ca/articles/2015/05/24/empowerment-comes-knowledge-your-heart-your-health.

1. The First Signs

1. S. O'Donnell et al., "Slow-Onset Myocardial Infarction and Its Influence on Help-Seeking Behaviors," *Journal of Cardiovascular Nursing* 27, no. 4 (August 2012): 334–44.

2. S. Dey et al., "Acute Coronary Syndromes: Sex-related Differences in the Presentation, Treatment and Outcomes among Patients with Acute Coronary Syndromes: The Global Registry of Acute Coronary Events," *Heart* 95, no. 1 (2009): 20–26.

3. Ibid.

4. Ibid.

5. Women's Heart Foundation, "Women and Heart Disease Facts," last modified 2007, http://www.womensheart.org/content/heartdisease/heart_disease_facts.asp.

6. *Heart Sisters* (blog), https://.myheartsisters.org/2009/08/14/how-does-it-feel/.

7. J. C. McSweeney, "Women's Early Warning Symptoms of Acute Myocardial Infarction," *Circulation* 108 (November 3, 2003): 2619–23.

2. Deadly Delay

1. B. Sherwood, "What It Takes to Survive a Crisis," *Newsweek,* January 23, 2009.

2. Ibid.

3. A. Rosenfeld et al., "Understanding Treatment-Seeking Delay in Women with Acute Myocardial Infarction: Descriptions of Decision-Making Patterns," *American Journal of Critical Care* 14, no. 4 (July 2005): 285–93.

4. L. Gould, email to the author, September 3, 2010.

5. WomenHeart: The National Coalition for Women with Heart Disease, "Support Networks," last modified 2016, http://www.womenheart.org/?page=SupportServices.

6. L. Steffel-Dennis, email to the author, September 5, 2014.

7. S. Hayes, "2000 Health Archetype Study: Hierarchy of Female Concerns," presented at WomenHeart Science and Leadership Symposium, Mayo Clinic, Rochester, Minnesota, October 11, 2008.

8. K. Hodgson et al., "Pets' Impact on Your Patients' Health: Leveraging Benefits and Mitigating Risk," *Journal of the American Board of Family Medicine* 28, no. 4 (2015): 526–34.

9. J. Yoder, "Finding Optimal Functioning in a Sexist World: A Social Justice Challenge," *Counseling Psychologist* 40 (2012): 1172–80.

3. Finally, a Correct Diagnosis

1. L. Mosca et al., "National Study of Physician Awareness and Adherence to Cardiovascular Disease Prevention Guidelines," *Circulation* 111 (2005): 499–510.

2. J. H. Pope et al., "Missed Diagnoses of Acute Cardiac Ischemia in the Emergency Department," *New England Journal of Medicine* 342, no. 16 (2000): 1163–70.

3. G. Chiaramonte, "Gender Bias in the Diagnosis, Treatment, and Interpretation of CHD Symptoms," paper presented at the Cardiovascular Research Foundation's 20th annual Transcatheter Cardiovascular Therapeutics (TCT) scientific symposium, Washington, D.C., October 12–17, 2008.

4. S. Laxmi et al., "Acute Myocardial Infarction in Women: A Scientific Statement from the American Heart Association," *Circulation* (January 25, 2016). http://circ.ahajournals.org/content/early/2016/01/25/CIR.0000000000000351.

5. L. Haywood-Cory, personal communication, May 1, 2011.

6. S. Hayes, email to the author, June 14, 2009.

7. S. Dey et al., "Acute Coronary Syndromes: Sex-related Differences in the Presentation, Treatment and Outcomes among Patients with Acute

Coronary Syndromes: The Global Registry of Acute Coronary Events," *Heart* 95, no. 1 (2009): 20–26.

8. Institute for Clinical Systems Improvement, Diagnosis and Treatment of Chest Pain and Acute Coronary Syndrome (ACS), Agency for Healthcare Research and Quality, National Guideline Clearing House, NGC:009521, revised November 2012.

9. C. N. Bairey Merz, "The Single Biggest Health Threat Women Face," *TEDxWomen* video, December 2011, http://www.ted.com/talks/noel_bairey_merz_the_single_biggest_health_threat_women_face?language=en.

10. S. Hayes, email to the author, January 22, 2010.

11. L. Mosca et al., "Evidence-Based Guidelines for Cardiovascular Disease Prevention in Women," *Circulation* 109, no. 5 (2004): 672–93.

12. N. Goldberg, *Women Are Not Small Men: Life-Saving Strategies for Preventing and Healing Heart Disease in Women,* New York: Ballantine, 2002.

13. Editorial, *Chicago Tribune,* "Only Male Subjects in Basic Science Research? Not Anymore," December 22, 2015.

14. M. Garcia, V. M. Miller, M. Gulati, S. N. Hayes, J. E. Manson, N. K. Wenger, C. N. Bairey Merz, R. Mankad, A. W. Pollak, J. Mieres, J. Kling, and S. L. Mulvagh, "Focused Cardiovascular Care for Women," *Mayo Clinic Proceedings* 91, no. 2 (February 2016): 226–40.

15. B. Goldman, "Doctors Make Mistakes. Can We Talk about That?," November 2011, *TEDxToronto* video, https://www.ted.com/talks/brian_goldman_doctors_make_mistakes_can_we_talk_about_that?language=en#.

16. Institute of Medicine, Report on Improving Diagnosis in Health Care, September 22, 2015.

17. R. Wachter, "Perspectives on Safety," interview with P. Croskerry, Agency for Healthcare Research and Quality, Patient Safety Network, May 2, 2010, https://psnet.ahrq.gov/perspectives/perspective/87.

18. M. Allen, "On the Surgeon's Scorecard," presentation at Medicine X conference, Stanford University, Palo Alto, CA, September 25, 2015.

4. The New Country Called Heart Disease

1. S. Westphal, "Pregnancy Problem Is a Heart Warning," *New York Times,* March 17, 2009.

2. L. Mosca et al., "Effectiveness-Based Guidelines for the Prevention of Cardiovascular Disease in Women—2011," *Circulation* 123 (March 21, 2011): 1243–62.

3. H. M. Dalal et al., "Cardiac Rehabilitation," *British Medical Journal* 351 (September 29, 2015), doi: https://doi.org/10.1136/bmj.h5000.

4. R. Arena et al., "Increasing Referral and Participation Rates to Outpatient Cardiac Rehabilitation: The Valuable Role of Healthcare Professionals in the Inpatient and Home Health Settings," *Circulation* 125 (January 30, 2012): 1321–29.

5. S. Hayes, response via Twitter to "The Surprising Reasons Heart Patients Don't Go to Cardiac Rehab," *Heart Sisters* (blog), April 7, 2015, https://myheartsisters.org/2015/04/05/why-heart-patients-dont-go-to-cardiac-rehab/.

6. J. Beckerman, *Heart to Start*, Portland, OR: Providence Heart and Vascular Institute, 2015.

7. B. Lown, "The Coronary Artery Entrapment," *Dr. Bernard Lown's Blog*, posted July 31, 2012, https://bernardlown.wordpress.com/2012/07/31/the-coronary-artery-entrapment/.

8. W. Sotile, *Heart Illness and Intimacy: How Caring Relationships Aid Recovery*, Baltimore: Johns Hopkins University Press, 1992.

9. R. Estruch et al., "Primary Prevention of Cardiovascular Disease with a Mediterranean Diet," *New England Journal of Medicine* 368 (April 4, 2013): 1279–90.

10. Mayo Clinic website, Healthy Lifestyle / Adult Health, "Denial: When It Helps, When It Hurts," May 20, 2014, http://www.mayoclinic.org/healthy-lifestyle/adult-health/in-depth/denial/art-20047926.

11. M. Katz, presentation at Medicine X conference, Stanford University, Palo Alto, CA, October 10, 2013.

12. P. Alsén, E. Brink, and L.-O. Persson, "Living with Incomprehensible Fatigue after Recent Myocardial Infarction," *Journal of Advanced Nursing* 65, no.5 (2008): 459–68.

13. M. Haykowsky et al., "A Meta-analysis of the Effects of Exercise Training on Left Ventricular Remodeling Following Myocardial Infarction: Start Early and Go Longer for Greatest Exercise Benefits on Remodeling," *Trials* 12 (April 4, 2011).

14. M. Jetté et al., "Metabolic Equivalents (METs) in Exercise Testing, Exercise Prescription, and Evaluation of Functional Capacity," *Clinical Cardiology* 8 (August 13, 1990): 555–65.

15. Ibid.

16. J. H. Mitchell et al., "The Exercise Pressor Reflex: Its Cardiovascular Effects, Afferent Mechanisms, and Central Pathways," *Annual Review of Physiology* 45 (October 1983): 229–42.

17. S. Fox, "Medicine 2.0: Peer-to-Peer Healthcare," *Pew Research Center*, September 18, 2011, http://www.pewinternet.org/2011/09/18/medicine-2-0 -peer-to-peer-healthcare/.

18. S. Laxmi et al., "Acute Myocardial Infarction in Women," *Circulation*, published online before print, January 25, 2016, http://circ.ahajournals.org /content/early/2016/01/25/CIR.0000000000000351.

19. *Heart Sisters* (blog), http://www.myheartsisters.org.

20. S. Fox, "Medicine 2.0: Peer-to-Peer Healthcare," *Pew Research Center.*

5. Depressing News about Depression and Heart Disease

1. S. Parker, email to the author, June 4, 2009.

2. E. Aletta, "Five Tips for Living Well with Chronic Illness," *Explore What's Next* (blog), July 19, 2010, http://explorewhatsnext.com/5-rules-for -living-with-chronic-illness/.

3. L. K. Bauer et al., "Effects of Depression and Anxiety Improvement on Adherence to Medication and Health Behaviors in Recently Hospitalized Cardiac Patients," *American Journal of Cardiology* 109, no. 9 (May 1, 2012): 1266–71.

4. C. Norris et al., "Depression Symptoms Have a Greater Impact on the 1-Year Health-Related Quality of Life Outcomes of Women Post–Myocardial Infarction Compared to Men," *European Journal of Cardiovascular Nursing* 6, no. 2 (June 2007): 92–98.

5. S. Mallik et al., "Depressive Symptoms after Acute Myocardial Infarction: Evidence for Highest Rates in Younger Women," *Archives of Internal Medicine* 166, no. 8 (2006): 876–83.

6. R. A. Bell et al., "Suffering in Silence: Reasons for Not Disclosing Depression in Primary Care," *Annals of Family Medicine* 5 (September–October 2011): 439–46.

7. S. Hayes, lecture to WomenHeart Science and Leadership Symposium for Women with Heart Disease, Mayo Clinic, Rochester, MN, October 2005.

8. D. Hare et al., "Depression and Cardiovascular Disease: A Clinical Review," *European Heart Journal* 35, no. 21 (2014): 1365–72.

9. J. Perk et al., "European Guidelines on Cardiovascular Disease Prevention in Clinical Practice," *European Heart Journal* 33, no. 13 (2012): 1635–701.

10. C. Norris et al., "Depression Symptoms Have a Greater Impact on the 1-Year Health-Related Quality of Life Outcomes of Women Post–Myocardial Infarction Compared to Men."

11. Island Heart to Heart: A seven-week series of educational lectures for recently-diagnosed heart patients and their family members in Victoria, B.C., Canada, presented by the non-profit Victoria Cardiac Rehabilitation Society, http://islandhearttoheart.ca/index.html.

12. WomenHeart: The National Coalition for Women with Heart Disease, "WomenHeart's Online Support Community," support group on Inspire .com, http://www.womenheart.org/default.asp?page=SupportServices.

13. WomenHeart: The National Coalition for Women with Heart Disease, "Support Services," http://www.womenheart.org/?page=Support _Networks.

14. S. Hayes, lecture to WomenHeart Science and Leadership Symposium for Women with Heart Disease, Mayo Clinic, Rochester, MN, October 2008.

15. S. Patten et al., "Clinical Guidelines for the Management of Major Depressive Disorder in Adults," *Journal of Affective Disorders* 117 (August 21, 2009): S26–S43, doi: 10.1016/j.jad.2009.06.041.

16. J. A. Blumenthal et al., "Exercise and Pharmacotherapy in the Treatment of Major Depressive Disorder," *Psychosomatic Medicine* 69, no 7 (2007): 587–96.

17. K. Salmansohn, "This Tool Saved Me from Depression," *Not Salmon* (blog), October 23, 2016, http://notsalmon.com/2016/10/23/tool-saved-me -depression/.

18. A. Child et al., "Meeting the Psychological Needs of Cardiac Patients: An Integrated Stepped-Care Approach within a Cardiac Rehabilitation Setting," *British Journal of Cardiology* 17 (July 2010): 175–96.

19. R. A. Bell et al., "Suffering in Silence: Reasons for Not Disclosing Depression in Primary Care," *Annals of Family Medicine*.

20. *Toronto Star*, February 12, 2013. https://www.thestar.com/news/gta /2013/02/12/clara_hughes_i_want_to_erase_the_stigma_of_mental _health_issues.html.

6. I'm What a Person with an Invisible Illness Looks Like

1. C. Miserandino, "The Spoon Theory," *But You Don't Look Sick* blog, June 1, 2003, https://butyoudontlooksick.com/articles/written-by-christine /the-spoon-theory/.

2. A. Becker-Schutte, "Hi There, Mr. Elephant— Let's Talk about Health Stigma and Privilege," *Dr. Ann Becker-Schutte* (blog), April 5, 2013, http://www.drannbeckerschutte.com/2013/04/hi-there-mr-elephant-lets-talk-about-health-stigma-privilege/.

3. K. Kastner, Twitter communication to the author, April 10, 2013.

4. L. B. Russell and M. A. Safford, "Time Requirements for Diabetes Self-Management: Too Much for Many?," *Journal of Family Practice* 54, no. 1 (2005): 52–56.

5. V. Montori, "Careful and Kind Care of Complex Patients," presentation to Maine Chronic Disease Improvement Collaborative learning session, Portland, ME, October 22, 2015, https://www.youtube.com/watch?v=WwywVtTyKJk.

6. M. Carl, V. Montori, and F. Mair, "We Need Minimally Disruptive Medicine," *British Medical Journal (BMJ)* 339 (August 11, 2009): 2803.

7. V. Montori and Mayo Clinic KER Unit, "The Instrument for Patient Capacity Assessment (ICAN)," *Minimally Disruptive Medicine* (website), October 5, 2015, https://minimallydisruptivemedicine.org/ican/.

8. WomenHeart: The National Coalition For Women With Heart Disease, http://www.womenheart.org/.

9. R. Moore and M. Chester, "Neuromodulation for Chronic Refractory Angina," *British Medical Bulletin* 59, no. 1 (2001): 269–78.

10. L. Steffel-Dennis, email to the author, September 5, 2014.

11. I. B. Mauss et al., "Don't Hide Your Happiness. Positive Emotion Dissociation, Social Connectedness, and Psychological Functioning," *Journal of Personality and Social Psychology* 100, no.4 (April 2011): 738–48.

12. B. Scott and C. Barnes, "A Multilevel Field Investigation of Emotional Labor, Affect, Work Withdrawal, and Gender," *Academy of Management Journal* 54, no. 1 (February 2011): 116–36.

13. Ibid.

14. L.Yanek et al., "Effect of Positive Well-Being on Incidence of Symptomatic Coronary Artery Disease," *American Journal of Cardiology* 112, no. 8 (2013): 1120–25.

7. One-Downmanship: You Think *You* Have Pain?

1. B. Keddy, "Fibromyalgia, Goodism, Self-Sacrifice, Giving Yourself Away," *Women and Fibromyalgia* (blog), May 9, 2009, http://womenandfibromyalgia.com/2009/05/09/fibromyalgia-goodism-self-sacrificegiving-yourself-away/.

2. S. Nolen-Hoeksema, "Rethinking Rumination," *Perspectives on Psychological Science* 3, no. 5 (September 2008): 400–424.

3. S. Nolen-Hoeksema, presentation to the American Psychological Association, Board of Scientific Affairs, Annual Convention, Washington, DC, August 19, 2005.

4. Ibid.

5. S. Taylor et al., "Biobehavioral Responses to Stress in Females: Tend-and-Befriend, Not Fight-or-Flight," *Psychological Review* 107, no. 3 (July 2000): 411–29.

6. S. Nolen-Hoeksema, "Rethinking Rumination," *Perspectives on Psychological Science.*

7. The Cleveland Clinic Cardiology Board Review, Lippincott Williams & Wilkins, 2012, Ch 46: 843.

8. R. N. Khouzam et al., "A Heart with 67 Stents," *Journal of the American College of Cardiology* 56, no. 19 (2010): 1605.

9. S. Hayes et al., "Familial Spontaneous Coronary Artery Dissection: Evidence for Genetic Susceptibility," *Journal of the American Medical Association Internal Medicine* 175, no. 5 (March 2015): 821–26.

10. S. Gilboa et al., "Congenital Heart Defects in the United States," *Circulation* 134 (July 2016): 101–9.

11. K. Keller and L. Lemberg, "Prinzmetal's Angina," *American Journal of Critical Care* 13 (July 2004): 350–54.

12. C. N. Bairey Merz et al., "Coronary Microvascular Dysfunction: Sex-Specific Risk, Diagnosis, and Therapy," *Nature Reviews Cardiology* 12 (May 2015): 406–14.

13. E. Creagan, "Going The Distance: Recognizing That Life Is Unfair," Mayo Clinic Healthy Lifestyle Stress Management, March 20, 2013, http://www.mayoclinic.org/healthy-lifestyle/stress-management/expert-blog/life-is-unfair/bgp-20056039.

14. R. Tedeschi and L. Calhoun, "Post-traumatic Growth: Conceptual Foundations and Empirical Evidence," *Psychological Inquiry* 15, no. 1 (2004): 1–18.

15. J. Gruman, "The Lemon of Illness and the Demand for Lemonade," *CFAH Prepared Patient Forum,* April 13, 2011, http://www.cfah.org/blog/2011/the-lemon-of-illness-and-the-demand-for-lemonade.

16. Ibid.

17. B. Ehrenreich, *Guardian,* January 2, 2010.

18. N. Stordahl, "Cancer Is Not a Gift," *Nancy's Point* (blog), December 12, 2011, http://nancyspoint.com/is-cancer-a-gift/.

19. K. Drum, *Mother Jones*, October 3, 2016.

20. T. M. Thrash and A. J. Elliot, "Inspiration as a Psychological Construct," *Journal of Personality and Social Psychology* 84, no. 4 (2003): 871–89.

21. M. Brown and J. Bussell, "Medication Adherence: WHO Cares?," *Mayo Clinic Proceedings* 86, no. 4 (2011): 304–14.

22. K. Teo et al., "Prevalence of a Healthy Lifestyle among Individuals with Cardiovascular Disease in High-, Middle- and Low-Income Countries: The Prospective Urban Rural Epidemiology (PURE) Study," *Journal of the American Medical Association* (April 17, 2013): 1613–21.

23. S. Reiser, "What Modern Physicians Can Learn from Hippocrates," *Cancer: Ethics and Law in Oncology* 98, no. 8 (October 2003): 1555–58.

24. http://www.goodreads.com/author/quotes/149539.Arthur_Ashe.

25. J. Jin et al., "Factors Affecting Therapeutic Compliance: A Review from the Patient's Perspective," *Therapeutics and Clinical Risk Management* 4, no. 1 (February 2008): 269–86.

8. On Being a Good Patient

1. R. Moore and M. Chester, "Neuromodulation for Chronic Refractory Angina," *British Medical Bulletin* 59, no. 1 (2001): 269–78.

2. D. Frosch et al., "Authoritarian Physicians and Patients' Fear of Being Labeled 'Difficult' among Key Obstacles to Shared Decision Making," *Health Affairs* 31, no. 5 (2012): 1030–38.

3. Ibid.

4. S. Mamede et al., "Do Patients' Disruptive Behaviours Influence the Accuracy of a Doctor's Diagnosis? A Randomised Experiment," *BMJ Quality and Safety*, published online, March 7, 2016, https://www.ncbi.nlm.nih.gov/pubmed/26951795.

5. *New York Times*, May 31, 2012.

6. L. Engelen, "The Origins of Patients Included," *Patients Included* (blog), https://patientsincluded.org/.

7. K. Lyons, "Cancer Charity Fundraiser Kate Granger Dies, Aged 34," *Guardian*, July 25, 2016.

8. K. Granger, personal communication in response to *Heart Sisters* blog article, "The Lost Art of Common Courtesy in Medicine," March 29, 2014,

https://myheartsisters.org/2011/12/27/the-lost-art-of-common-courtesy
-in-medicine/.

9. M. Kahn et al., "Etiquette-Based Medicine," *New England Journal of Medicine* 358, no. 19 (2008): 1988–89.

10. S. Tackett et al., "Appraising the Practice of Etiquette-Based Medicine in the Inpatient Setting," *Journal of General Internal Medicine* 28, no. 7 (2013): 908–13.

11. K. O'Leary et al., "Hospitalized Patients' Understanding of Their Plan of Care," *Mayo Clinic Proceedings* 85, no. 1 (2010): 47–52.

12. I. Brook, "A Laryngectomy Shakes This Physician to the Core," *Kevin MD* (blog), January 19, 2011, http://www.kevinmd.com/blog/2011/01/laryngectomy-shakes-physician-core.html.

13. Ibid.

9. The New Normal

1. British Heart Foundation, "7 Most Common Heart Disease Myths," *Heart Matters* online journal, https://www.bhf.org.uk/heart-matters-magazine/medical/7-most-common-heart-disease-myths/?utm_medium=social&utm_source=twitter&utm_campaign=broadcast&utm_content=organic.

2. S. Moore, "The Cure Myth: Coronary Heart Disease," Massachusetts General Hospital (video), http://www.massgeneral.org/news/multimedia.aspx?id=250.

3. D. Kanzari, "Coronary Stents Do Not Improve Long-Term Survival," presentation to the American Heart Association scientific meeting, New Orleans, LA, November 7, 2004.

4. Ibid.

5. J. P. Erwin, Twitter conversation with the author, April 9, 2016.

6. P. Mitrou et al., "Mediterranean Dietary Pattern and Prediction of All-Cause Mortality in a US Population. Results from the NIH-AARP Diet and Health Study," *Archives of Internal Medicine* 167, no. 22 (2007): 2461–68.

7. J. Mandrola, *Dr. John M* (blog), http://www.drjohnm.org/.

8. P. Cirillo and B. Cohn, "Pregnancy Complications and Cardiovascular Disease Death: Fifty-Year Follow-Up of the Child Health and Development Studies Pregnancy Cohort," *Circulation* 132, no. 13 (September 29, 2015): 1234–42, doi: CIRCULATIONAHA.113.003901.

9. C. D. Fryar et al., "Prevalence of Uncontrolled Risk Factors for Cardiovascular Disease: United States, 1999–2010," *NCHS Data Brief,* No. 103, 2012.

10. R. Hambrecht et al., "Percutaneous Coronary Angioplasty Compared with Exercise Training in Patients with Stable Coronary Artery Disease: A Randomized Trial," *Circulation* 109 (March 8, 2004): 1371–78.

11. S. Möbius-Winkler et al., "Coronary Collateral Growth Induced by Physical Exercise," *Circulation* 133 (2016): 1438–48.

12. C. Thomas, "Learning to Love Your Open Heart Surgery Scar," *Heart Sisters* (blog), October 26, 2012, https://myheartsisters.org/2012/10/26/love-your-scars/.

13. H. Marano, "The Art of Resilience," interview with S. Wolin, *Psychology Today*, May 1, 2003.

14. J. Jackson, "Five Years Post-STEMI," *Skinny Bitch Chronicles* (blog), October 2, 2016, https://skinnybitchchronicles.com/2016/10/02/five-years-post-stemi/.

15. L. Berk et al., "Cortisol and Catecholamine Stress Hormone Decrease Is Associated with the Behavior of Perceptual Anticipation of Mirthful Laughter," presented at the 121st Annual Meeting of the American Physiological Society, San Diego, CA, April 5, 2008.

16. WomenHeart: The National Coalition of Women with Heart Disease, online support community forum topic: "You Know You Have Heart Disease When . . . ," *Inspire*, December 6, 2010, https://www.inspire.com/groups/womenheart/.

17. C. Thomas, "Stupid Things That Doctors Say to Heart Patients," *Heart Sisters* (blog), January 13, 2011, https://myheartsisters.org/2011/01/13/stupid-things-doctors-say-heart-patients/.

18. K. Neff, *Self-Compassion* (blog), www.selfcompassion.org.

19. Ibid.

20. Ibid.

10. Making Peace with an Errant Organ

1. V. Roger et al., "Heart Disease and Stroke Statistics—2012 Update: A Report from the American Heart Association, *Circulation* 125, no. 1 (2012): 2–220.

2. K. Sharma and M. Gulati, "Coronary Artery Disease in Women: A 2013 Update," *Global Heart* 8, no. 2 (2013): 105–12.

3. J. Jackson, "Post–Heart Attack Stun," guest post in *My Life in Red* (blog), February 25, 2013, http://www.mylifeinred.net/heart-attack-stun/.

4. Ibid.

5. "Captain Phillips" (film), *Wikipedia*, last modified October 25, 2016, https://en.wikipedia.org/wiki/Captain_Phillips_(film).

6. Editorial, "When Denial Can Be Harmful," *Mayo Clinic Healthy Lifestyle Adult Health*, May 20, 2014, http://www.mayoclinic.org/healthy-lifestyle /adult-health/in-depth/denial/art-20047926?pg=2.

7. K. Charmaz, "Loss of Self: A Fundamental Form of Suffering in the Chronically Ill," *Sociology of Health and Illness* 5, no. 2 (1983): 168–97.

8. Ibid.

9. Ibid.

10. Ibid.

11. Ibid.

12. Ibid.

13. Ibid.

14. Ibid.

15. Ibid.

16. Anonymous, emailed comment to the author via *Heart Sisters* (blog), June 22, 2011, http://www.myheartsisters.org.

17. S. Nuland, "How We Die: Is It Improving or Not?," Ernest Becker Foundation presentation, Kane Hall, University of Washington, Seattle, WA, July 28, 2011, https://www.youtube.com/watch?v=H89MC3xHZO0.

18. "Coping with Feelings," American Heart Association, http://www .heart.org/HEARTORG/Conditions/More/CardiacRehab/Coping-with -Feelings_UCM_307092_Article.jsp#.V_q5ktw7TnE, April 22, 2014.

19. J. Prokopy, "How Do I Deal with Anger at My Chronic Illness?," *Chronic Babe* (blog), January 22, 2014, http://www.chronicbabe.com/awap -wednesday-how-do-i-deal-with-anger-at-my-chronic-illness/.

20. J. Thorson, "Get Checked: Women's Risk Factors for Heart Disease," *My Life in Red* (blog), February 14, 2015, http://www.mylifeinred.net/wo mens-risk-factors-for-heart-disease/.

21. S. Lyubomirsky, "The Science of Happiness," lecture at Pepperdine University, Seaver College, W. David Baird Distinguished Lecture Series, Malibu, California, September 25, 2014, https://www.youtube.com/watch ?v=pliMc1eO_34.

22. Ibid.

23. C. Wallis, "The New Science of Happiness," *Time*, January 9, 2005, http://content.time.com/time/magazine/article/0,9171,1015832-4,00.html.

Carolyn's Patient-Friendly, Jargon-Free Glossary of Confusing Cardiology Terms

Like any exclusive club, heart disease has its own shorthand jargon, understandable only by other members of the club, particularly by our cardiac care providers. This is why heart patients often need a translator.

After my heart attack, I wanted to learn as much as I could about what the heck had just happened to me. I Googled the simple question, "Why did my left arm hurt during my heart attack?" Dr. Google led me to a California-based site called *HealthTap*. At first blush, the site looks like a free Q&A service for patients' questions that real doctors (complete with head shots and full CVs) will answer. It's one of a growing number of online matchmaking services between patients looking for doctors and doctors wanting to expand their practices. But sure enough, there was a question listed on the site, identical to mine. Here's how the cardiac surgeon answering this question responded to the heart patient who asked it: "The pericardium is innervated by C3,4,5 (phrenic nerve). There may be some neuronal connections to the intercostobrachial nerves."

If you understood that gobbledygook, you don't need my glossary. But for the rest of us, here's a plain-English translation of some of the most common acronyms/terms/abbreviations you're likely to find on your own chart or around the cardiac ward.

ablation (or cardiac ablation): an invasive procedure to scar or destroy specific tissues in the heart that can trigger an abnormal heart rhythm.

ACE inhibitor (angiotension converting enzyme inhibitor): a drug used in the treatment of high blood pressure or heart failure. It helps to relax the blood vessels, prevent scar formation, improve heart function, and reduce mortality in patients diagnosed with heart failure or heart attack.

acute coronary syndrome (ACS): an emergency condition brought on by sudden reduced blood flow to the heart muscle. The first sign of acute coronary syndrome can be sudden stopping of your heart (cardiac arrest).

AED (automatic external defibrillator): a portable defibrillator used on patients experiencing sudden cardiac arrest by applying a brief shock to the heart through electrodes placed on the chest.

angina (stable): a condition marked by predictable and manageable cardiac symptoms such as chest pain or other symptoms typically felt between neck and navel that come on with exertion but go away with rest. Angina is caused by an inadequate blood supply to the heart muscle, and managed by resting or using medication like nitroglycerin. Emotional stress, hot or cold weather, eating a big meal, or smoking can also aggravate stable angina.

angina (unstable): a more serious condition, occurring when blood flow through a narrowed coronary artery is severely blocked. The pain of unstable angina is not relieved by rest; it's a medical emergency and requires immediate attention.

angiography: a technique of injecting a dye into an artery in the wrist or groin, with x-ray guidance, to help outline the heart and coronary blood vessels. An angiogram is a test that can help doctors identify blockages, narrowing, or abnormalities in the coronary arteries. *See also* angioplasty; cardiac catheterization

angioplasty: an invasive but non-surgical technique for treating diseased arteries by temporarily inflating a tiny balloon inside an artery during angiography. A tiny metal stent is usually inserted during this procedure to help keep the artery propped open. Also called percutaneous coronary intervention (PCI).

anti-platelet drugs: medications that block the formation of blood clots by preventing the clumping of platelets (e.g., Plavix, Effient, Brillinta, Ticlid, etc.); often prescribed to patients with stents, usually combined with daily low-dose aspirin.

aorta: the main artery of the body, carrying blood from the left side of the heart to the arteries of all limbs and organs except the lungs.

aortic stenosis: a heart valve problem in which the opening of the aortic valve is narrowed.

aortic valve: one of four valves in the heart, this valve allows blood from the left ventricle to be pumped up (ejected) into the aorta, and prevents blood from returning to the heart once it's in the aorta.

apex: the lowest bottom tip of the heart; it points downward at the base.

arrhythmia: a condition in which the heart beats with an irregular or abnormal rhythm.

ASA: generic form of aspirin.

atherosclerosis: a condition in which the plaque building up inside arteries affects their ability to carry oxygen-rich blood to the heart muscle and other parts of your body. Plaque is made up of fat, cholesterol, calcium, and other substances found in the blood, and can narrow the coronary arteries, reducing blood flow to your heart muscle and increasing the risk of blood clots.

atrial fibrillation or Afib: an irregular and often rapid heart rate that can cause poor blood flow to the body. *See also* paroxysmal atrial fibrillation

atrial flutter: an irregular or abnormal heart rhythm in which the upper chambers of the heart (atria) beat very fast, causing the walls of the lower chambers (ventricles) to beat inefficiently as well.

atrium: a collecting chamber of the heart that receives blood from the body or lung veins before the blood enters the pumping chamber (the ventricle); plural is atria.

beta blocker (BB): a drug that can improve mortality and reduces recurrent heart attack in patients diagnosed with coronary artery disease or heart failure; also limits the activity of epinephrine, a hormone that increases blood pressure.

bicuspid aortic valve (BAV): the most common malformation of the heart valves, in which the aortic valve has only two cusps instead of three.

BID: medication instructions—two times a day (in Latin, "bis in die").

blood pressure (BP): the force or pressure exerted by the heart in pumping blood; the pressure of blood in the arteries. *See also* hypertension

blood thinners: drugs used to prevent the formation of blood clots. Blood thinners don't really thin the blood, but they help to prevent it from clotting.

BMI (body mass index): a BMI number can tell you if you are overweight. A BMI higher than 30 is considered obese. Here's the three-step formula to determine your own BMI number: multiply your weight in pounds by 703, then multiply your height in inches by itself, and finally, divide the figure from step 1 by the figure in step 2. Or simply Google *BMI Calculator* for a quick and easy way to do this calculation online.

BPM: beats per minute (how fast the heart is beating). The normal heart rate in the average adult ranges from 60–100 beats per minute.

broken heart syndrome: a heart condition that is not a heart attack, but feels like one, with common symptoms such as severe chest pain and shortness of breath. It often follows a significant emotional stress. Also known as Takotsubo cardiomyopathy, stress cardiomyopathy, stress-induced cardiomyopathy, and apical ballooning syndrome.

Brugada syndrome (BrS): a genetic heart disease that puts patients at increased risk of sudden cardiac arrest, identified by distinctively abnormal EKG test results.

bundle branch block or BBB: a condition in which parts of the heart's electrical system are defective, causing an irregular heart rhythm (arrhythmia).

bypass surgery (CABG or coronary artery bypass graft): surgery that reroutes blood flow around a diseased blood vessel in the heart by grafting either a piece of vein from the leg or a piece of artery from under the breastbone.

CABG: (pronounced "cabbage"; *see* bypass surgery).

calcium channel blocker: a drug that lowers blood pressure by regulating calcium-related electrical activity in the heart.

cardiac arrest (or sudden cardiac arrest): the stopping of the heart, usually because of interference with the electrical signal (often associated with coronary heart disease). Can lead to sudden cardiac death if the heart is not restarted.

cardiac catheterization (PCI): an invasive procedure in which a catheter is inserted through a blood vessel in the wrist/arm or groin, with x-ray guidance. This procedure can help provide information about blood supply through the coronary arteries, blood pressure, blood flow throughout the chambers of the heart, collection of blood samples, and x-rays of the heart's ventricles or arteries. It's performed in the cath lab. *See also* angiography; angioplasty

cardiac output: the amount of blood the heart pumps through the circulatory system in one minute.

cardiac resynchronization therapy (CRT): also called a bi-ventricular pacemaker, an electronic pacing device that's surgically implanted in the chest to treat an irregular heartbeat.

cardiac tamponade: pressure on the heart that occurs when blood or fluid builds up in the space between the heart muscle (myocardium) and the outer covering sac of the heart (pericardium).

cardiomyopathy: a chronic disease of the heart muscle (myocardium), in which the muscle is abnormally enlarged, thickened, and/or stiffened.

cardioversion: a medical procedure in which an abnormally fast heart rate (tachycardia) or cardiac arrhythmia such as atrial fibrillation is converted to a normal rhythm using an electric current or drugs.

catheter: a very long thin tube inserted into an artery or vein in your wrist/arm or (mostly in the US) the groin, and threaded through blood vessels up to the heart during angiography.

cath lab: the room in the hospital / medical facility where cardiac catheterization procedures take place (for example, when a stent is implanted into a blocked coronary artery). *See also* angioplasty

CCU (Coronary Care Unit): the intensive care ward for heart patients with severe cardiac problems and/or recuperating from cardiac surgery.

cholesterol: a waxy, fat-like substance that's found in all cells of the body, and in some foods we eat. Your body needs cholesterol to make hormones, vitamin D, and substances that help you digest foods. Sometimes these fatty plaque deposits can build up within your coronary arteries. If you've been told you have high cholesterol, it probably means that you have higher levels of LDL (low-density lipoprotein, or bad) cholesterol, which may mean you're at higher risk of getting coronary heart disease. But if you have high amounts of HDL (high-density lipoprotein, or good) cholesterol in your blood, your risk of getting heart disease may be lower. Your physician will look at the blood test numbers that reflect your total cholesterol.

cognitive behavioral therapy (CBT): a type of talk therapy recommended for heart patients, helping people change their patterns of thinking, which can then help to change the way they feel.

collateral arteries: extra coronary blood vessels that are sometimes able to bypass a blockage in an artery in order to supply enough oxygenated blood to enable the heart muscle to survive during a heart attack.

congenital heart defect: any of about 35 different types of heart conditions that occur in about 1 percent of live births, when a baby's heart or blood vessels near the heart don't develop normally before the baby is born. Because of medical advances in treatment of babies born with heart defects, there are now for the first time more adults living with congenital heart disease than children.

coronary artery disease (CAD): a narrowing of the arteries that supply blood to the heart, caused by a plaque rupture, blood clot, or spasm; greatly increases the risk of a heart attack.

coronary microvascular disease: a heart condition that causes impaired blood flow to the heart muscle through the smallest blood vessels of the heart. Also called microvascular disease (MVD) or small vessel disease.

coronary reactivity test: an angiography procedure specifically designed to examine how blood vessels in the heart respond to different medications. Physicians use these images to distinguish among different types of blood vessel dysfunction (e.g., coronary microvascular disease).

costochondritis: a cause of severe chest pain that is not heart related; it's a very painful inflammation of the cartilage that connects a rib to the breastbone. In New Zealand, physiotherapists treat their costo patients with specific back exercises and massage; in North America, we use anti-inflammatory drugs.

Coumadin: a brand-name drug taken to prevent the blood from clotting and to treat blood clots. Coumadin is prescribed to reduce the risk of blood clots causing strokes or heart attacks. *See also* warfarin

CP (chest pain): a cardiac symptom that may also be felt as squeezing, pressure, fullness, pressure, heaviness, burning, or tightness. It's the most commonly experienced symptom of heart attack in both men and women, but at least 10 percent of women report no chest symptoms at all during their heart attacks.

CPR (cardiopulmonary resuscitation): an emergency procedure in which the heart and lungs are made to work by manually compressing the chest overlying the heart, sometimes along with forcing air into the lungs, used to maintain circulation when the heart stops pumping during cardiac arrest. Current guidelines suggest hands-only CPR. *See also* AED

CV (cardiovascular): pertaining to the heart and/or blood vessels that make up the circulatory system.

diastolic blood pressure: the blood pressure measured in the arteries when the heart muscle is relaxed between beats. Example: the second number, if your blood pressure reading is 120/80.

dilated cardiomyopathy: a disease of the heart muscle, primarily affecting the heart's main pumping chamber (left ventricle). The left ventricle becomes enlarged (dilated) and can't pump blood to your body with as much force as a healthy heart can.

diuretic: a class of drugs used to lower blood pressure. Also known as water pills.

Dressler's syndrome: this can happen to some people three to four weeks after a heart attack. The heart muscle that was damaged during the attack sets the immune system in motion, increasing antibodies that can attack the thin coverings of your heart or lungs. Chest pain is the most common symptom; often treated with anti-inflammatory drugs.

dual antiplatelet therapy (DAPT): medications that help to block the formation of blood clots by preventing the clumping of platelets, prescribed along with aspirin, especially to patients who have had a stent implanted (examples: Plavix, Effient, Brillinta, Ticlid, etc.).

echocardiogram: a test to measure how the heart is functioning using ultrasound waves to produce a visual display, used for the diagnosis or monitoring of heart disease; a stress echocardiogram adds an exercise component to make the heart beat faster before the echocardiogram is recorded.

ectopic beats: small changes in a heartbeat that is otherwise normal, leading to extra or skipped heartbeats.

EF (ejection fraction): a measurement of the percentage of blood pumped out of the left ventricle with each heartbeat. The normal measurement is about 55–70 percent. Your ejection fraction can be measured during an echocardiogram, nuclear medicine tests, cardiac catheterization, or a cardiac MRI.

EKG (electrocardiogram or ECG): a test in which several sticky sensors are placed on the body to monitor the electrical activity of the heartbeat. In some countries, it's called an ECG.

endothelium: a single-cell layer of flat endothelial cells lining the closed internal spaces of the body, such as the inside of blood vessels. Endothelial dysfunction affects the ability of these cells to help dilate blood vessels, control inflammation, and prevent blood clots. The endothelium is associated with most forms of cardiovascular disease, such as hypertension, coronary artery disease, chronic heart failure, peripheral vascular disease, diabetes, chronic kidney failure, and severe viral infections.

enhanced external counterpulsation (EECP): a non-invasive, non-drug treatment for angina. It works by promoting the development of collateral coronary arteries and is widely used in prominent heart clinics such as the Cleveland Clinic, Mayo Clinic, and Johns Hopkins, especially for patients who may not be good candidates for invasive procedures such as bypass surgery, angioplasty, or stents.

EP (electrophysiologist): a cardiologist who has additional training in diagnosing/treating electrical or heart rhythm disorders.

ER (Emergency Room): the part of the hospital where people in need of emergency medical care are treated. Also called the ED (Emergency Department) or the A & E (Accident and Emergency) department.

exercise stress test: a diagnostic test typically ordered to look for the presence of coronary artery disease. This can be performed either by having a person exercise or by giving medications that mimic the effects of exercise on the heart. The effect of the exercise on blood flow is then assessed either by EKG, echocardiogram, or nuclear imaging. *See also* MIBI; nuclear stress test; stress echocardiography

familial hypercholesterolemia (FH): a genetic tendency to have dangerously high cholesterol levels in the blood. FH is an inherited disorder that can lead to aggressive and premature cardiovascular disease, including heart attacks, strokes, or narrowing of the heart valves.

GERD (gastroesophageal reflux disease): a chronic digestive condition that occurs when stomach acid or, occasionally, stomach content, flows back into your esophagus (food pipe), irritating its lining. Also called acid reflux or heartburn. Because some GERD symptoms (such as chest pain) often mimic heart attack symptoms, heart patients can sometimes be misdiagnosed, as I was, with GERD.

HDL (high density lipoprotein): a component of blood cholesterol, HDL helps protect against heart disease by promoting cholesterol breakdown and removal from the blood; hence, its nickname, good cholesterol.

heart attack (myocardial infarction or MI): damage to an area of the heart muscle (myocardium) resulting from a blocked blood supply to that area. The part of the heart muscle fed by that blocked artery no longer receives enough blood and oxygen to work properly. After a heart attack, scar tissue may form in the damaged muscle. In some cases, the remaining heart muscle has to work harder to pump blood throughout the body.

heart failure (formerly known as congestive heart failure): a weakness of the heart in which the heart has trouble pumping all the blood it needs to. This can lead to a backup of blood in the blood vessels and an accumulation of fluid in the body's tissues, including in the lungs.

Holter monitor: a portable monitoring device that patients wear for recording heartbeats over a period of 24 hours or more.

hypertension (HTN): high blood pressure, or the force of blood pushing against the walls of arteries as it flows through them.

hypertrophic cardiomyopathy (HCM): a heart condition that damages the muscle wall of the lower chambers of the heart and causes them to thicken abnormally. HCM is perhaps best known as a leading cause of sudden cardiac death in young athletes.

ICD (implantable cardioverter defibrillator): a surgically implanted device designed to recognize certain types of abnormal heart rhythm (arrhythmia) and correct them in case of erratic heartbeats or sudden cardiac arrest.

inappropriate sinus tachycardia (IST): a heart condition seen most often in young women in which a person's resting heart rate is abnormally high (greater than 100 bpm), their heart rate increases rapidly with minimal exertion, and this rapid heart rate is accompanied by symptoms of palpitations, fatigue, and inability to exercise.

INR (international normalized ratio): a lab test measurement of blood coagulation, often used as a standard for monitoring how well anticoagulant drugs such as warfarin (Coumadin) are working.

interventional cardiologist: a cardiologist with specialized training to diagnose and treat cardiovascular disease as well as congenital (present at birth) and structural heart conditions by performing catheter-based procedures such as angioplasty and stenting.

ischemic heart disease (IHD): heart problems caused by narrowing of the coronary arteries, causing a decreased blood supply to the heart muscle. Also called coronary artery disease or coronary heart disease.

IVUS or intravascular ultrasound: a form of echocardiography in which a tool called a transducer is threaded into the heart blood vessels via a catheter; it's used to provide detailed information about blockages inside the coronary arteries. *See also* left anterior fascicular block; right bundle branch block

KER Unit: the Knowledge and Evaluation Research Unit at Mayo Clinic, a laboratory focused on translating best available research evidence into clinical practice, led by Dr. Victor Montori.

LDL (low density lipoprotein): the body's primary cholesterol-carrying molecule. High blood levels of LDL may increase your risk of heart disease by promoting cholesterol attachment and accumulation in blood vessels; often called "bad cholesterol."

left anterior descending (or LAD) coronary artery: one of the heart's coronary artery branches from the left main coronary artery, which supplies blood to the left ventricle.

left anterior fascicular block (LAFB): an abnormal condition of the left ventricle of the heart, related to, but distinguished from, left bundle branch block. *See* left bundle branch block.

left bundle branch block: a heart rhythm problem (arrhythmia) in which the electrical impulses along a specific pathway within the heart muscle cause your heart to beat abnormally.

left circumflex artery: this artery carries freshly oxygenated blood from the heart to the body; it's a branch of the left main coronary artery.

left main coronary artery: the artery that branches from the aorta to supply freshly oxygenated blood to the heart via the left anterior descending artery (LAD) and the left circumflex artery.

Lipoprotein-a or Lp(a) (pronounced "L P little a"): a high level of Lp(a) molecules made of proteins, cholesterol, and similar substances in the blood is considered a risk factor for heart disease; it's detectable with a specific blood test.

long QT syndrome: a heart rhythm disorder that can cause fast, chaotic heartbeats that may trigger a sudden fainting spell or seizure. In some cases, the heart may beat erratically for so long that it can cause sudden death.

LOS: length of stay (that patients remain hospitalized).

lumen: the hollow area within a tube, such as inside a blood vessel. You may hear statements like "deposits of plaque narrowed the lumen of the artery."

LVAD (left ventricular assist device): a mechanical device that can be placed outside the body or implanted inside the body. An LVAD helps the heart pump oxygen-rich blood from the left ventricle to the rest of the body, usually while the patient is waiting for a heart transplant.

main pulmonary artery: carries oxygen-depleted blood from the heart to the lungs to get re-oxygenated there.

MI (myocardial infarction, or heart attack): damage to an area of the heart muscle (myocardium) resulting from a blocked blood supply to that area. The part of the heart muscle fed by that blocked artery no longer receives enough blood and oxygen to work properly. After a heart attack, scar tissue may form in the damaged muscle. The remaining heart muscle may then have to work much harder to pump blood throughout the body.

MIBI (cardiac perfusion scan or nuclear stress test): a test used to assess blood flow to the heart muscle while it's being stressed by exercise or medication, to find out what areas of the heart muscle have decreased blood flow due to coronary artery disease. A tiny amount of a chemical that emits a type of radioactivity called gamma rays is injected into a vein in the arm or hand to perform this test.

microvascular disease (MVD, coronary microvascular disease, or small vessel disease): a heart condition of the smallest blood vessels that results in impaired blood flow to the heart muscle. Symptoms mimic those of a heart attack.

mitral valve (MV): one of four valves in the heart, this structure controls blood flow between the heart's left atrium (upper chamber) and left ventricle (lower chamber). The mitral valve has two flaps (cusps).

mitral valve prolapse: a condition that occurs when the leaflets of the mitral valve between the left atrium (upper chamber) and left ventricle (lower chamber) bulge into the atrium and permit backflow of blood into that chamber of the heart. The condition is often associated with progressive mitral regurgitation.

mitral valve regurgitation (also called mitral insufficiency or mitral incompetence): failure of the mitral valve to close properly, causing blood to flow back into the heart's upper left chamber (the left atrium) instead of moving forward into the lower left chamber (the left ventricle).

mitral valve stenosis: a narrowing of the mitral valve that may result from an inherited (congenital) problem or from rheumatic fever.

MRI (magnetic resonance imaging): a non-invasive diagnostic test using strong magnetic fields and radio waves to form pictures of the body.

MUGA (multiple-gated acquisition scanning): a non-invasive nuclear heart test that uses a radioactive isotope called technetium to evaluate how the heart's ventricles are functioning.

murmur: heart noises that can be heard alongside normal heart sounds. They are caused by congenital defects or damaged heart valves that do not close properly and allow blood to leak back into the originating heart chamber.

myocardial infarction (MI, heart attack): damage to an area of the heart muscle (myocardium) resulting from a blocked blood supply to that area. The part of the heart muscle fed by that blocked artery no longer receives enough blood and oxygen to work properly. After a heart attack, scar tissue may form in the damaged muscle. The remaining heart muscle may have to work much harder to pump blood throughout the body.

myocardium: the muscular tissue of the heart.

nitroglycerin (or nitro): a type of nitrate medication that helps to relax and dilate arteries; often used to prevent/treat the chest pain of angina; taken when needed or available in long-acting nitrate patches or ointments. Also called NTG or GTN.

normal sinus rhythm (NSR): the characteristic rhythm of the healthy human heart. NSR is considered to be present if the heart rate is in the normal range, the P waves are normal on the EKG/ECG, and the heart rate does not vary significantly.

NSTEMI (non-ST-segment-elevation myocardial infarction): a heart attack identical to unstable angina except that cardiac enzymes are also elevated. NSTEMI heart attack is a type of acute coronary syndrome that does not produce an ST-segment elevation on an electrocardiogram test (EKG/ECG). It's usually associated with a severely blocked coronary artery, limiting blood flow to the heart muscle in that area. *See also* STEMI

nuclear stress test: a diagnostic test that usually involves two exercise stress tests, one while you're exercising on a treadmill or stationary bike with isotopes like thallium or other radioactive dyes injected into your bloodstream, and another set while you're at rest. A nuclear stress test is used to gather information about how well your heart works during physical activity and at rest. *See also* MIBI; thallium stress test

open heart surgery: a surgical procedure in which the chest is opened up and surgery is performed on the heart muscle, valves, coronary arteries, or other parts of the heart. *See also* bypass surgery

pacemaker: a surgically implanted electronic device that helps regulate the heartbeat.

palpitations: a noticeably rapid, strong, or irregular heartbeat due to agitation, exertion, or illness.

paroxysmal atrial fibrillation: this type of atrial fibrillation lasts from a few seconds to days. There are often no clear triggers to these atrial fibrillation episodes.

PCI (percutaneous coronary intervention, or angiography): procedures performed in the cardiac catheterization laboratory (cath lab). Angioplasty and stenting the coronary artery are examples of PCI. Also called a percutaneous transluminal coronary angioplasty (PTCA).

pericardium: the outer covering sac of the heart.

peripheral artery disease: a common circulatory problem in which narrowed arteries reduce blood flow to the limbs, usually to the legs. Women living with PAD may actually have few if any symptoms or present with atypical symptoms, but ironically are more functionally impaired, with either reduced walking distance or speed, than men are. The leg pain of PAD when walking is known as claudication.

plaque: a deposit of fatty substances that may form on the inner lining of the artery wall, characteristic of atherosclerosis.

post-op (postoperative): the period of time after surgery.

post-partum cardiomyopathy (PPCM): a form of cardiomyopathy that causes heart failure toward the end of pregnancy or in the months immediately after delivery, in the absence of any other cause of heart failure.

POTS (postural orthostatic tachycardia syndrome): a disorder that causes an increased heart rate and low blood pressure, which can lead to light-headedness and sometimes fainting spells when a person stands up.

preeclampsia: elevation of the blood pressure during late pregnancy, typically associated with protein in the urine. This can increase a woman's future risk of heart disease.

Prinzmetal's variant angina: chest pain caused by a spasm in a coronary artery that supplies blood to the heart muscle. *See also* vasospasm

PRN: medication instructions—as needed (from the Latin "pro re nata," meaning "as the circumstance arises"), used when medications are prescribed to be taken not at specified times, but only when and if you need them.

prodromal: referring to one or more very early symptoms that might indicate the start of a medical problem before the patient is actually aware that something serious is happening. See more on early warning signs of a heart attack that are frequently reported by female survivors in chapter 1.

PTCA (percutaneous transluminal coronary angioplasty): *See* angioplasty.

pulmonary valve: one of the four valves in the heart. Located between the pulmonary artery and the right ventricle of the heart, it helps to move blood toward the lungs and keeps it from sloshing back into the heart.

pulmonary vein (PV): a vein carrying freshly oxygenated blood from the lungs to the left atrium of the heart.

PVC (premature ventricular contraction): an early or extra heartbeat that happens when the heart's lower chambers (the ventricles) contract too soon, out of sequence with the normal heartbeat.

QID: medication instructions—four times a day. The Latin is "quater in die."

restenosis: the re-narrowing of an artery after stent placement. Sometimes called stent failure.

rheumatic heart disease: a condition causing damage to the valves of the heart due to repeated attacks of rheumatic fever.

right atrium: the upper right chamber of the heart, a collecting chamber of the heart that receives blood from the body or lung veins before the blood enters the pumping chamber (the ventricle), which then sends blood to the lungs to be oxygenated.

right bundle branch block (RBBB): a delay or obstruction along the pathway that electrical impulses travel to the right side of the heart to make it beat. *See also* left bundle branch block

right coronary artery: the artery that supplies oxygenated blood to the right side of the heart.

right main coronary artery: the artery that supplies oxygenated blood to the walls of the heart's ventricles and the right atrium.

right ventricle: the lower right chamber of the heart; it receives deoxygenated blood from the right atrium and pumps it into the lungs via the pulmonary artery.

SAD: seasonal affective disorder, a light-related condition that can aggravate feelings of depression.

SCAD: spontaneous coronary artery dissection (see below).

septal defect: a hole in the wall of the heart separating the atria (two upper chambers of the heart) or in the wall of the heart separating the ventricles (two lower chambers).

sestamibi stress test: *see* MIBI.

sick sinus syndrome: a heart rhythm disorder that is typically composed of a tachycardia (fast heart rhythm, or atrial fibrillation) alternating with bradycardia (slow heart rhythm, or heart block).

sinus bradycardia: abnormally slow heartbeat.

sinus node (or sinoatrial node): a small bundle of nerve cells situated in the upper part of the wall of the right atrium (the upper right chamber of the heart) where the heart's electrical impulses are generated. It's the normal natural pacemaker of the heart and is responsible for initiating the heartbeat.

sinus tachycardia: a heart rhythm greater than 100 beats per minute (bpm) in an average adult. The normal heart rate in the average adult ranges from 60–100 bpm. Also called sinus tach or sinus tachy.

SOB: shortness of breath.

spasm: *see* vasospasm.

spontaneous coronary artery dissection (SCAD): an emergency condition that occurs when a tear forms in one of the blood vessels in the heart, causing a heart attack, abnormalities in heart rhythm, and/or sudden death. SCAD tends to strike young healthy women with few if any cardiac risk factors, particularly during pregnancy or the post-partum period, or women with fibromuscular dysplasia, a condition that causes narrowing (stenosis) or enlargement (aneurysm) of the arteries.

statins: any of a class of drugs that lower the levels of low-density lipoproteins (LDL)—the bad cholesterol in the blood. Examples of brand name statins: Lipitor, Crestor, Zocor, Mevacor, Levachol, Lescol, etc.

STEMI: the more severe form of the two main types of heart attack. A STEMI (or ST-elevation myocardial infarction) is usually caused by a sudden complete (100 percent) blockage of an artery feeding the heart muscle. A non-STEMI (or NSTEMI) is a heart attack usually caused by a severely narrowed artery, not necessarily completely blocked.

stenosis: a narrowing of a passage in the body (e.g., caused by a blockage inside a coronary artery).

stent: a tiny implantable device made of expandable metal mesh (looks a bit like a tiny chicken-wire tube) that is placed using a balloon catheter at the site of a narrowing coronary artery during an angioplasty procedure. The stent is then expanded inside the artery by inflating the tiny balloon and left in place to help keep the artery open. The coronary stent was named after Charles Stent (1807–1885), an English dentist whose real claim to fame occurred when he suggested using a material he invented to coat underwater trans-Atlantic cables, which had broken several times as a result of corrosion by seawater.

stint: a common spelling mistake if what you really mean is the word *stent*. See above.

stress echocardiography: a standard echocardiogram test that's performed while a person exercises on a treadmill or stationary bicycle. This test can be used to visualize the motion of the heart's walls and pumping action under stress to check how well the heart is able to pump blood. The echocardiogram is performed just before and just after the exercise part of the procedure.

stress test: a diagnostic test typically ordered to look for the presence of coronary artery disease. This can be performed either by having a person exercise or by giving medications that mimic the effects of exercise on the heart. The effect of the exercise on blood flow is then assessed either by EKG/ECG, echocardiogram, or nuclear imaging. *See also* exercise stress test; MIBI; nuclear stress test; stress echocardiography

sudden cardiac arrest: the complete stopping of the heartbeat, usually because of interference with the electrical signal (often associated with coronary heart disease). Can lead to sudden cardiac death.

systolic blood pressure: the highest blood pressure measured in the arteries. It occurs when the heart contracts with each heartbeat. Example: the first number in a blood pressure reading of 120/80.

tachycardia: abnormally fast heart rate, at least 100 beats per minute (bpm).

Takotsubo cardiomyopathy: a heart condition that can mimic a heart attack. It is not a heart attack, but it feels just like one, with common symptoms such as severe chest pain and shortness of breath. It often follows a severe emotional stress. Also referred to as broken heart syndrome, stress cardiomyopathy, stress-induced cardiomyopathy or apical ballooning syndrome.

TAVR (transcatheter aortic valve replacement): a minimally invasive procedure to repair a damaged or diseased aortic valve. A catheter is inserted into an artery in the groin and threaded to the heart. A balloon at the end of the catheter, with a replacement valve folded around it, delivers the new valve to take the place of the old. Also called TAVI (transcatheter aortic valve implantation).

thallium stress test: thallium is one of a number of possible radioactive dyes used in a stress test. *See also* nuclear stress test

TIA (transient ischemic attack): a stroke-like event that lasts only for a short time and is caused by a temporarily blocked blood vessel feeding the brain.

TID: medication instructions—three times a day. The Latin is "ter in die."

transesophageal echocardiogram (TEE): this test involves an ultrasound transducer inserted down the throat into the esophagus, in order to take clear images of the heart structures without the interference of the lungs and chest.

transthoracic echocardiogram (TTE): this is the standard echocardiogram, a painless test similar to an x-ray but without the radiation, using a hand-held device called a transducer placed on the chest to transmit sound waves (ultrasound). These sound waves bounce off the heart structures, producing images and sounds that can be used by the doctor to detect heart damage and disease.

treadmill test (or exercise stress test): a common heart test while walking/running on a treadmill or pedaling a stationary bike to make your heart work harder and beat faster. An EKG/ECG is recorded while you exercise to monitor any changes in your heart under stress, with or without the aid of drugs to enhance the test. *See also* echocardiogram; MIBI; nuclear stress test

tricuspid valve: one of four one-way valves in the heart; a valve with three little flaps that keeps blood in the right ventricle from flowing back into the right atrium. *See also* valves

triglycerides (Tg): the most common fatty substance found in the blood, normally stored as an energy source in fat tissue. High triglyceride levels may make a person more susceptible to clot formation. High triglyceride levels tend to accompany high LDL (bad) cholesterol levels and other risk factors for heart disease.

valves: your heart has four one-way valves that keep blood flowing in the right direction. Blood first enters the heart through the tricuspid valve, and next goes through the pulmonary valve (sometimes called the pulmonic valve) on its way to the lungs. Then the freshly oxygenated blood returning from the lungs passes through the mitral valve and leaves the heart through the aortic valve.

vasodilator: a drug, such as nitroglycerin, that causes blood vessels to dilate.

vasospasm: a coronary artery spasm that can cause severe chest pain and sudden constriction of the blood vessel, reducing its diameter and blood flow to the heart muscle. *See also* Prinzmetal's variant angina

ventricle: each of the two main lower chambers of the heart, one called the left and one called the right.

ventricular bigeminy: a heart rhythm condition in which the heart experiences two beats of the pulse in rapid succession.

ventricular fibrillation (VF): a condition in which the ventricles (two lower chambers of the heart) contract in a very rapid, unsynchronized fashion. When fibrillation occurs, the ventricles cannot pump blood throughout the body. Most sudden cardiac deaths are caused by VF or ventricular tachycardia (VT or VTach).

warfarin: a generic drug taken to prevent the blood from clotting and to treat existing blood clots. Warfarin is believed to help reduce the risk of blood clots causing strokes or heart attacks. Also known as Coumadin (brand name).

widow maker heart attack: the type of heart attack I survived, a nickname doctors use to describe a severely blocked left anterior descending (LAD) coronary artery, or the left main coronary artery that directly feeds the LAD. The widow maker term is used because, if the blockage happens high enough near the beginning of the artery, it can deprive a large area of the heart muscle immediately below that blockage of any oxygenated blood flow. All heart attacks are serious, but the consequences of the widow maker are often catastrophic, because the heart muscle damage may be large enough to lead to sudden cardiac death. Please note the gender imbalance here: despite the number of women like me who do experience this type of heart attack, doctors still aren't calling this the widower maker.

Wolff-Parkinson-White syndrome (WPW): a heart condition in which an extra electrical pathway connects the atria (two upper chambers) and the ventricles (two lower chambers), causing a rapid heartbeat.

Index